The Birds and the Bees Guide to

Allergy-Free Living

Scott E. Seargeant
Seargeant Publishing Company, Inc.

As individuals (mentally, physically and genetically) we respond differently to external forces. Keep this in mind when using this book. As indicated, this is a guide and is not represented as an exact science or to be true to everyone. Because of our individuality, a few people may be allergic to some of the plants considered allergy-free or low pollen producers. However, in general population terms, the plants represented in this guide are categorized correctly. The phrase allergy-free and low pollen producer are used interchangeably in this book.

Copyright © 1997

Printed in the United States of America by Jostens Printing and Publishing.
For information address: Seargeant Publishing Company, Inc.,
P.O. Box 1849, Visalia, CA 93279

— Library of Congress Cataloging-in-Publication Data —
Allergy-Free Living: The Birds and the Bees Guide to
by Scott E. Seargeant - 1st. ed.
ISBN - 0-9657867-0-6

Cover designed by Scott E. Seargeant and Lesley D. Gleason
Cover photographs by Trudy Johnson Photography

FIRST EDITION

To my son Kyle,

and to all parents and children who
suffer from allergies and asthma

FOREWORD

Pollen counts and warnings for people who suffer from allergies to remain indoors are common announcements across the United States. Many doctor visits for both children and adults are due to allergy symptoms and the misery that accompanies them. Since there is no real cure for allergies, relief is achieved through treatment of the symptoms with medicines, and prevention strategies. Many people who don't currently suffer from allergy symptoms will have these problems in the future because of repeated exposure to allergens such as pollen. Indoor air conditioning and air filters provide relief only while indoors. Once the allergic person steps outdoors, he or she is again assaulted by the allergens in the air.

Eliminating or drastically reducing the allergens we are exposed to by using allergy-free plants in landscaping around our homes and businesses is an ideal way to improve our health. Allergy sufferers will have less symptoms due to reduced exposure to the allergens, and potential allergy sufferers may be able to avoid developing symptoms altogether. Scott Seargeant's book is an excellent tool to help all of us achieve this goal. It is written in layman's terms to educate us about the growing allergy problem caused by allergy producing plants and gives a practical guide to eliminate the problem. Medical professionals, allergy sufferers and concerned parents will all benefit from the information provided. Working together we can reduce, if not eliminate a major health problem without damaging our environment.

Dr. of Pediatric and Adolescent Medicine   Susan M. Caldwell M.D.,
                                                                               F.A.A.P.

FOREWORD

Sneezeless landscaping is more than whimsical fantasy, it's an issue critical to our health. It addresses America's number one environmental hazard, pollution. Yellow rain is pollen pollution and to us the worst of all pollutants. The pollen count escalates yearly. It emanates from trees, grasses and weeds. Man is an inadvertent victim intercepting the pollen with his nose before it can otherwise reach and propagate plants. Twenty percent of Americans suffer the consequences of pollen pollution termed Hay Fever! It's like a cold that won't quit lasting on the average of nineteen weeks! Symptoms vary from blocked noses, teary eyes, and unnerving itching, to such complications as sinusitis, headaches, ear infections, bronchitis, and asthma. Costs run into the billions.

Some communities have gone so far as outlawing highly-allergenic plants. Las Vegas, Neveda and Tuscon, Arizona have had such restrictions. Bermuda grass, mulberry and olive trees have been targeted. One year after these restrictions, the grass pollen count dropped 50 percent. A different approach exists in Fresno and Visalia, California. Both cities have developed "demonstration gardens" exhibiting the beauty and fragrance of low allergy plantings. They were devised and designed to provide a model of what residential and public housing, school grounds, nurseries, parks, shopping malls, street divides, and freeway linings should be to issue good health and safety to its citizens.

Scott Seargeant has always been one of the strong leaders in this movement. He was the designer of the Visalia project 12 years ago. His guide is sorely needed. Were it reasonably followed, our "quality of life" (physical, social and mental health) would have improved dramatically. This book should be required reading for the City Fathers, planning departments, landscape designers, contractors, nurserymen, school administrators, and John Q. Public. Hats off to you, Scott, for writing among the best of "How to Books."

Dr. of Allergy and Respiratory Medicine   William H. Ziering M.D.
Central California Research Institue

ACKNOWLEDGMENTS

Many people have contributed ideas and information during the writing of this book. In appreciation of their efforts, I would like to acknowledge them.

Dr. William Ziering, Allergist. Devoted to the eradication of allergies. Developer of the Allergy-Free Gardens.

Chuck Duncan, Certified Arborist. An experienced and knowledgeable arborist. Chuck introduced me to the idea of allergy-free plants.

Dennis Lipson, Entrepreneur. A man of great knowledge and kind heart who always seemed to have the right answer when I needed one.

Dave Rice, Computer Consultant. He always kept me online and updated.

My wife Colleen, and children Kyle, David, and Brianne for their help, support, and understanding.

Mr. Boething and Jeff Pierson, Boething Tree Land Nursery. For allowing me to take photos of their nursery stock.

Trudy Johnson, Photographer. For her professional excellence and enthusiasm in photographing the cover.

Lesley Gleason, Marketing Consultant. A gifted person. Designer of the cover, editor, and marketing specialist.

CONTENTS

CONTENTS Con't.

PREFACE

The purpose of this book is to identify the plants around your home, office and community that are allergy producing and replace them with allergy-free or low pollen producing plants. I do not advocate removing heritage or beautiful specimen trees just because they are allergy producing. However, if allergy producing plants around your yard, office and community are not functionally, aesthetically or historically important, then I suggest they be removed and replaced with allergy-free plants.

Reducing allergies by removing the plants that cause allergy symptoms will make a big difference. Like many things, it all starts at home.

— Scott E. Seargeant

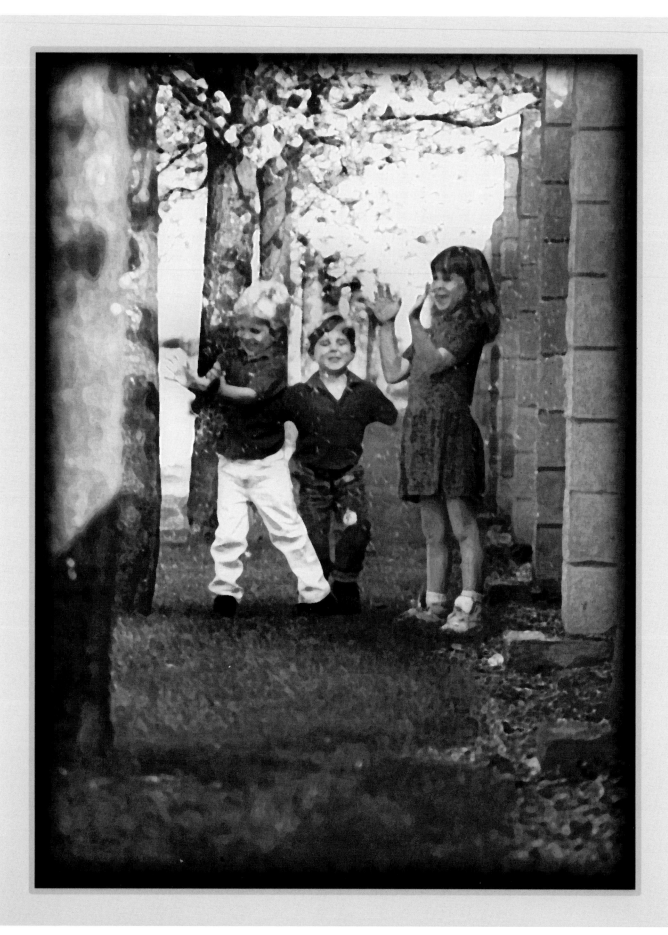

*I*ntroduction

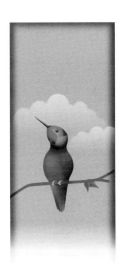

"In the years to come the number of people reported to have allergies will increase significantly. The amount of pollen from different sources will inundate our noses, throats and lungs. The need to educate the public now on planting plants that are low pollen producers or allergy-free is immense."

I wrote this in 1987 for a speech at a ribbon cutting ceremony for the opening of the largest allergy-free park in the United States of America. Little did I know the time would come so soon. Allergy producing plants are being planted without regard to human health. As these allergy plants mature they begin to spew billions of tiny pollen grains into the atmosphere waiting to be inhaled.

Those who do not currently have allergies could care less about the things that don't concern or bother them. However, some of these people are walking allergy time bombs waiting to go off, unknowing that at any time their bodies could react negatively to the pollen in their system. For some it's just a matter of time. Time for new neighborhood allergy plants to grow bigger and produce more pollen, or time for the allergy producing ash, olive, or mulberry trees they planted in their yard to mature and thus produce a hefty dose of pollen. Of course, the allergy producing plants at the office are not exempt from your lungs either. They too can be affecting your immune system. Add a little stress from work or home and pow you become symptomatic, you become allergic, now you start to care! You start to think planting those allergy producing ash, olive and mulberry trees wasn't such a good idea after all, and maybe you should have planted a fescue lawn instead of an allergy provoking bermuda lawn. It doesn't seem so important now that you don't have to mow your bermuda lawn in the winter.

Then you start to think of your children. Are they going to become allergic too! You begin to panic. Where can I find information on the plants that do and don't cause allergies? Bits and pieces of information are available but the definitive knowledge you desperately seek can't be found.

To some this scenario may sound silly. If it does, then you probably have never had plant allergies. To allergy sufferers it sounds all too familiar, until now. This book was written for you the allergy sufferer or for friends and family that suffer from allergies. I hope this book is used over and over again, helping people understand allergies, allergy-free and allergy producing plants, and how to start rearranging your outdoor environment. In hope that one day the allergy sufferer can really enjoy the great outdoors even if the great outdoors is in your own backyard.

Just in case there is a stigmatism concerning allergy-free plants that I am not aware of, then I would like to nip it in the bud. Allergy-free plants are real plants you see everyday, they just don't produce the quantities of pollen into the air needed to produce allergies or the pollen produced doesn't cause allergic reactions in people. Really, its that simple. Allergy-free plants are not like diet sodas or fat free food, they look like the real thing, because they are the real thing. The unsure and confident should read on and both will discover the real benefits of allergy-free living — increased quality of life.

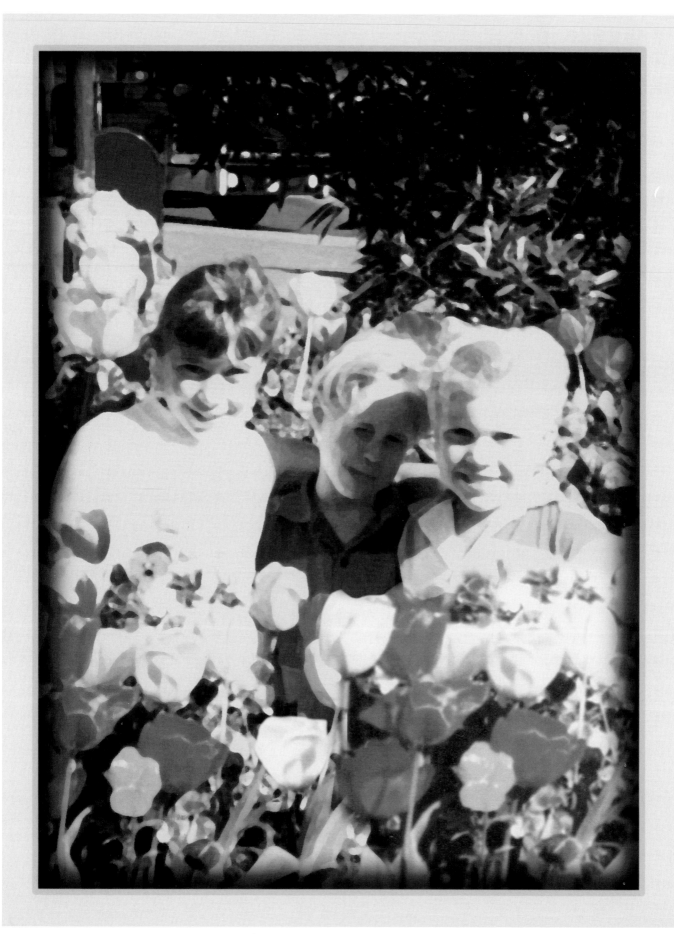

Chapter 1

Allergies

◣ *What is an Allergy ?*

An allergy, as defined in a dictionary, is "an exaggerated or abnormal reaction to substances, situations or physical states harmless to most people." An allergist's definition, in simple terms, is "a reaction to a harmless material." The important word in any definition of an allergy is "harmless." The substance causing an allergy must be a normally harmless material to other people, and yet, even in small amounts affects the allergic person. An extremely dusty wind or a smoke-filled room would tend to cause most anyone to sneeze, cough or have watery eyes. This type of reaction is not considered to be an allergy simply because it could happen to anyone. However, if mowing your lawn or walking by a specific species of plant material causes you to sneeze several times or break-out in hives, this would be considered an allergic reaction to a harmless material, and you would truly be "allergic" to those substances.

◣ *Allergy Population Statistics*

There are over 52 million allergy and asthma sufferers in the United States. Plant pollen is responsible for a major portion of these allergies. According to allergists, the pollen counts for Tucson, Arizona and Fresno, California have sky-rocketed. Pollen counts tripled from 1979 to 1986. Since then, pollen counts have been out of control. In the first week of March, 1996, 2.1 million people, mostly in the Southwest and West, were affected by seasonal allergies; an increase of 300,000 people from the previous year's figure of 1.8 million.

The impact allergies have on our health and wealth are staggering. The 1986 statistic for loss of wages from allergies was in excess of one billion dollars! Medical expenses for doctors, hospitals, and medicine reached 3 billion dollars. Asthma increased 70 percent from 1980 to 1989. The average number of allergy related fatalities (including asthma) tops 4,000 per year and is rising 8 percent a year! It was reported in June of 1992 that allergies (and asthma) cost patients nearly 5 billion dollars a year. This accounted for one out of very nine doctor visits.

Children are being hit hard by the increase in allergens. One out of very five visits to the pediatrician is allergy related. Children miss 10 million school days every year due to allergies, and it is the number one reason children miss school. The need to reduce allergies by reducing plants that cause allergies is unprecedented. The awareness of allergies and their symptoms has led to changes in diagnosis. Cold symptoms of spring and summer were further examined to find many sufferers actually had seasonal allergies.

Areas once considered to be havens for allergy sufferers, places like Phoenix and Tucson, Arizona, are now so inundated with pollen and pollution that they are actually heading the list of allergy producing cities. The city of Tucson, recognizing its allergy problems, passed ordinances limiting or restricting the use of certain allergy plants. The first year after enacting the ordinance, the pollen count dropped 50 percent. Hopefully, legislative acts like this will be our last resort. Voluntary planting of allergy-free or low pollen producing plants is the key. People in positions of influence, such as architects, landscape contractors, park superintendents, home owners, business owners, doctors, community, regional, state and federal leaders, need to recognize the serious impact allergies have on our society. Steps need to be taken. Easy steps. It all starts with education, so keep reading, and start acting.

◣ *How do People Become Allergic?*

Allergies are mostly inherited, that is, they are a function of your genetic makeup. The percent of potentially allergic people in the world is in somewhat of a dispute. Depending on the source it can range from 10 percent to as high as 50 percent or higher. A moderate and generally accepted figure is 25 percent. This means that approximately 25 percent of the people have the potential to produce the antibodies that can at some time cause them to have allergies. These types of people are said to be atopic. An atopic person may never show any symptom of an allergic reaction. The other 75 percent of the population "shouldn't" experience any allergies. It can be difficult to determine whether a person is allergy susceptible or allergy-free. The predictability of a genetic occurrence of allergies in children is undeterminable. This is partly due to the fact that allergies can skip generations.

The allergy sufferer or potential sufferer becomes symptomatic or allergic when his exposure levels, duration and intervals to allergen(s) become greater than the body's natural immune system can properly handle. At this point, the body reacts to the antigen, such as pollen, and produces chemical reactions that surface into allergic symptoms, like a runny nose or itchy eyes, nose, and throat. A person exhibiting an allergic reaction is said to be sensitized. Once a person becomes sensitized the battle is on and desensitizing "cures" are initiated.

◼ *The Longevity of Allergenic Conditions*

Because of the inherent nature of allergies, once you become an allergic person you will remain allergic the rest of your life. This does not mean you will carry the symptoms of your allergies the rest of your life; however, you will always carry the capacity to produce the antibodies that cause allergy symptoms. Lots of people outgrow their allergic symptoms but not their allergic condition. For example, children can outgrow their symptoms of hay fever only to acquire the symptoms of asthma later in life which in turn could subside and resurface into other allergic symptoms. Allergy symptoms do not occur in any definite cycle or pattern.

◼ *The Order of Allergic Reactions*

The first step in the allergenic process is the exposure to antigens such as pollen, mold, and cat dander. The antigens cause the production of antibodies. Antibodies are proteins in your body that fight foreign substances like pollen. When an adequate number of antibodies are produced, the antigen combines with the antibodies causing a union which releases certain chemical compounds, one of which is histamine.

Histamines are found in your body's cells, and under normal conditions perform useful functions. However, when a person is exposed to an antigen, an excess amount of histamine is produced causing the histamine to flow out of the cell and into the circulatory system. This excess amount of histamine can cause three fundamental responses including constriction, dilation, and seepage of fluid from blood vessels into the tissues. These fundamental responses are the causes of all allergic reactions throughout the body.

In order to combat symptoms of the "histamine" in their bodies many people take an "antihistamine." However, antihistamines are generally supposed to be taken before exposure to the antigens. A doctor should always be consulted before taking any medication(s).

Chapter 2

Medical Conditions Triggered by Allergies

◣ Hay Fever

Hay fever is one of the most common types of allergies today. The symptoms of hay fever are sneezing, runny nose, watery eyes, red and swollen eyes, itchy nose and eyes, itchy ears, and itchy palate. Occasionally this allergy is accompanied by a rash. These symptoms can range from slightly allergic to moderately allergic to severely allergic reactions.

Plant pollens are the major source of hay fever. Plants that cause hay fever produce millions of microscopic wind born pollen grains. The most harmful of which are trees, grasses and weeds. The first to cause major havoc are the deciduous trees in early spring. By late spring the grasses have revived themselves from winter layoff and are in full bloom. Later, in summer the weeds have matured to the point of reproduction and are spewing out millions upon millions of wind-born pollen.

Climatic conditions also play a big part in the severity of a person's allergies. More rain in spring and summer months will reduce the amount of pollen in the air and thus reduce the amount of contact a person would normally receive during these times. However, more spring and early summer rain will increase the number and size of weeds causing increased allergies in the late summer and early fall. Conversely, a dry or excessively windy spring or summer will increase the amount of pollen in the air and also the amount of exposure. There is more pollen in the air at dusk and early morning than at any other time.

Hay fever is most common with younger children, but can become a problem at any age.

◣ Allergic Rhinitis

The bulk of hay fever sufferers' problems arise from pollen and mold allergens. However, allergic rhinitis, more commonly known as the "stuffy nose syndrome," is caused by many different types of allergens including pollutants and irritants such as tobacco smoke, hair sprays, deodorants, perfumes, automobile exhaust, industrial pollution, insect repellents, and pesticides. Strong smells or odors including polishes, paints, ammonia and even cooking odors can be considered pollutants or irritants to a person suffering from allergic rhinitis.

Allergic rhinitis symptoms are similar to those caused by the hay fever allergens except that they can occur during anytime of the year or season. The symptoms include nasal stuffiness, runny nose, sneezing, sniffing, postnasal drip, and the inability to smell or tolerate certain odors. Some of the symptoms are worse in the morning. The symptoms are also worse indoors than they are outdoors.

◣ Sinusitis

Sinusitis is a condition specific to the upper respiratory system or what is referred to as the paranasal sinuses, and is caused by a combination of allergy and infection. These paranasal sinuses are actually pairs of air sacs located in the head and face area. There are several pairs of air sacs, the largest of which is the maxillary sinus located underneath the cheekbones. The other sinus air sacs are the frontal sinus located behind the eyebrows, and the ethmoid and sphenoid sinus air sacs which lie deeper in the head. All the sinuses are connected to the nose through tiny openings called ducts.

The sinuses' main function is to provide an extra supply or reservoir of air to the upper respiratory tract. This air reserve helps balance any change in pressure (as related to elevation changes) and also warms and humidifies incoming nasal air. They also reduce the weight of the head and play a big part in the tonal quality of the voice.

Sinusitis symptoms occur when the air sacs fill with mucous and prevent the sinus ducts from draining into the nose. This causes a feeling of fullheadedness, facial pains over one or both cheeks, headaches above the eyebrows, clogged or runny nose, voice changes, fever, a feeling of weakness or laziness, and the familiar postnasal drip.

There are two kinds of sinusitis: acute and chronic. Acute sinusitis is primarily caused by infection and usually responds favorably to a combination of antibiotics and decongestants. The symptoms will subside after a few days to a week. Chronic sinusitis is allergy based and needs further examination to determine the causal allergens.

Serous Otitis

Serous otitis is an ailment of the middle ear and is caused by a build-up of serous fluid in the middle ear cavity. Its symptoms are earaches and impaired hearing, and it is usually affiliated with some form of nasal allergy. Children are more prone to serous otitis than adults.

Asthma

Bronchial asthma is a disorder characterized by the recurring yet reversible exhibitions of wheezing. Asthma attacks the large and medium size air passages (bronchi) of the lung, causing inflammation and build-up of mucous in the respiratory tree.

Genetics play a big part in the occurrence of asthmatic people. The main causes of asthmatic attacks are inhalant allergens and infection. Emotion, physical activity, and environmental irritants are considered to be secondary causes.

Inhalant allergens of pollen and mold cause mostly seasonal occurrences of asthma. Asthma from infection can start anywhere in the respiratory tract. Viral infections are more common than bacterial infections. Asthma can also be triggered by the infectious drip of mucous into the lower respiratory tract caused by chronic sinusitis. Activity related asthma attacks are more likely to happen while jogging, snow skiing or playing basketball than while swimming, walking or playing golf. Emotion, as a secondary affiliate to asthma, usually occurs during times of high stress at home, school or work. Environmental or non-allergic irritants such as automobile exhaust, smoke, industrial pollutants, and paints all play havoc with the asthmatic person. Changes in the air quality, temperature, and humidity can also cause symptoms of asthma.

Chapter 3

Inhalant Allergens

Pollen

Pollen is the powdery male sexual reproductive cell produced from the anthers of a plant usually in association with a flower. Pollen is the main inhalant allergen. Other inhalant allergens include molds, animal dander, dust mites, and insect feces.

Almost all higher plants produce pollen. However, not all pollen causes allergic reactions. The main factors determining whether plant pollen is considered to be allergenic has to do with the capabilities of the pollen to position itself in the environment to significantly cause continual exposure to the potential allergy sufferer. Once a person is exposed, the pollen must be able to cause an allergenic reaction. So, in actuality, it's the exposure potential and allergenic reaction potential that generally helps determine a plant's (pollen) classification.

Classification

Generally speaking, there are two kinds of pollen, the kind that produces allergenic reactions in people and the kind that do not. The differences between the two stem from their physical properties and their distribution, quantities produced, and reactive qualities. After studying these different properties and qualities of various pollen, a distinctive pattern starts to develop enabling us to simplistically classify them into their respective groups. Basically, a plant that has the potential to cause allergenic reactions in people will produce massive amounts of light, powdery pollen that is naturally adapted to pollinate other flowers of the same species by way of the wind. This "wind-blown pollen," can travel from just a few feet to hundreds of miles depending on the wind patterns and velocities. A pollen of this nature can easily spread over a large area causing extensive exposure. Conversely, a plant that lacks the potential or opportunity to cause allergies will produce lower quantities of heavy, often sticky pollen, that is naturally adapted to pollinate other plants of the same species by way of animals and insects (birds and bees). This type of pollen is referred to as the insect or bird pollen. In this instance the pollen from these plants does not get the chance to come in contact with the allergy or potential allergy sufferer unless, of course, he or she sticks his or her nose into the flowers. But even then the pollen must be one that will cause an allergenic reaction.

In summary, if the pollen cannot easily and freely get into the environment, then it should have a hard time causing wide-spread allergenic reactions. As is in most cases, prevention (from exposure to allergens) is the best medicine.

Air Quality

The quality of the air we breath is continually decreasing. Auto and industry pollution coupled with dust and pollen, often cause health risks to the susceptible or sensitive. These people are warned to stay indoors and limit their outdoor travel on really bad air days. This is no way to live! Steps have been taken to reduce auto and industry pollution; however, very few steps have been taken to reduce allergy symptoms by reducing the causal agent, pollen, from allergy producing plants. There are several reasons for this. First of all, information on allergy-free and allergy producing plants has not been widely available (until now). Secondly, smoke and pollution can cause anyone to react negatively. Not everyone is allergic to pollen. Here lies a major distinction between allergy and pollution.

Curtailing pollution means becoming more energy efficient and or limiting your personal lifestyle. Curtailing allergy symptoms means planting allergy-free plants and removing non-essential allergy producing plants. Currently, unrestricted landscape planting choices limit the allergy sufferer's lifestyle. He/she is told to stay indoors and not to exert themself. In the meantime, he/she experiences a runny nose, itchy eyes, ears and throat; he/she can't breath easily and are tired, irritable, and so on. This is no way to live.

The most commonly used recommendation concerning allergy from pollen is to "avoid going outdoors when pollen counts are high." Most adults have to work, most children go to school. Just going from your front door to your car or traveling to work can be enough to cause allergy symptoms, especially if your immediate landscapes at home and work are producing allergy provoking pollen. Add to this a trip to the super market where the parking lot is filled with allergy producing trees and it's no wonder so many people are afflicted with allergy problems. Children walking or riding the school bus can be exposed to even higher amounts of pollen, especially when playing on the school grounds in or near allergy provoking plants.

The time has come to reduce allergy producing plants through allergy-free planting and by educating others to do the same. This recycling process will reduce the pollen in our lives and lead to a healthier lifestyle.

Chapter 4

Reducing the Allergy "Triggers"

◤ Reducing the Triggers

The first step in reducing each person's allergy symptoms is to identify the triggers (plants) that cause the allergic reactions. The easiest way is to consult your doctor or allergist. Either one can perform certain tests that indicate your susceptibility to a particular allergen. Generally, there will be several allergens that will trigger your symptoms. Once these plants are identified, you should decrease the length and frequency of exposures to them in your home, work, school, and community.

◤ Getting Started

The best way to reduce your allergy triggers is to rearrange your outdoor environments, first at home, then at work, and finally in your community. To accomplish this you must have a master plan. Start by leisurely flipping through the pages in the "Allergy-Free Plant" chapter and write down the plants that appeal to you. Then, look up each plant you have selected, noting the characteristics and requirements of each, such as the size, flower color, exposure, and water requirements. If you are inclined to landscape or re-landscape on your own then read below. If you do not have a green thumb then skip this section and go directly to "Hiring a Professional."

◤ The Do-It-Yourself Person

New Landscapes:

New landscape sites at home, office or community may not have existing plants. If not, there is no need to identify any allergy producing plants. In the case of allergy producing weeds, keep the site free by hoeing, tilling or spraying an appropriate weed killer. Weeds usually pollinate as they reach maturity so kill them early before they produce pollen.

Formulate a master plan by first studying the landscape site and listing as many of the characteristics as you can. Examples of these include geographic location, orientation of the sun, soil type, grade, utility locations, septic system/sewer lines, and easements. Next, design your landscape on paper locating hardscape elements like concrete driveways and walkways. Following this, select all the trees, shrubs, ground cover, grass, and flowers you need to design your landscape. Don't choose common bermuda lawns when deciding on a lawn grass. Bermuda grass is one of the worst allergy offenders.

Upon final selection of the allergy-free plants you would like to use in your landscape, note their characteristics and uses. Find appropriate place(s) on your design for each plant species selected and label them. You may select several plant choices for the same designated area on your design. An example would be selecting camellias, azaleas, rhododendrons, and ivy for a proposed shady area on the design. These four plants fit the requirements for a shady area, but you may only use one or two of them in the actual design. Two key elements in designing a landscape are placing the plants in the correct location according to their specific requirements, and using plants that accent, compliment, and contrast in an aesthetically, functionally, and thematically pleasing way. For example, pine and palm trees tend not to go together. Conversely, redwoods, fir or pine can be very appealing and give the landscape an alpine or mountain feeling (theme). Designing with a theme in mind can prevent thematic crossovers. Once your plan is in place, you can begin installing your landscape.

Existing Landscapes:

Check your landscape site and identify the plants in your yard that are allergy producing by using the information in Chapter 6 "Allergy Producing Plants." Determine the value of all allergy producing plants in your yard. For example, most shrubs, flowers, and ground cover can be replaced without totally changing the appearance of the landscape. The biggest change a landscape will have involves the trees and grass.

A well-manicured lawn can make or break the aesthetic appearance of a landscape. Replacing lawn with shrubs or ground cover is a good idea for several reasons, but is not always feasible. Changing the type of lawn in your landscape can be the best compromise provided the lawn is maintained regularly.

Whenever possible common bermuda grass should be replaced with a less pollen producing grass like fescue or hybrid bermuda. Most pollinating grasses cause some degree of allergy symptoms if they are allowed to set seed (pollinate). Fescue grass seems to be a good alternative when lawn grass is desired.

Trees can also change the look of a landscape dramatically. Removal of large trees can disrupt the ecology of the landscape and cause changes in plant microclimates. This can damage or kill some plants like dogwoods, cast-iron plants, azaleas, camellias, and rhododendrons. Conversely, it can improve other sun-loving plants that were gradually shaded out as the tree(s) grew larger, namely shrub daisy, flowering quince, rockrose, and crape myrtle.

Removal of any mature, healthy, structurally-sound tree should not be an easy decision. Mature viable trees have immense value. The removal of mature allergy producing trees should be weighed against the overall historical, functional and aesthetic value they may possess. However, any tree that is unhealthy or structurally weak should always be removed for safety purposes.

Small, insignificant, allergy producing trees should be removed and or replaced with appropriate allergy-free trees. The biggest quandry concerning the removal of an allergy producing tree will be the dissapearance of functional and aesthetic value, for example, shade and loss of proportion and scale in the landscape. This can be overcome, especially if it is accomplished over several years, by interplanting allergy-free trees near or around the allergy producing tree(s). As the allergy-free trees are increasing in size the allergy producing tree(s) need to be pruned proportionately to decrease their size. This cycle is repeated annually or semi-annually. Once the allergy-free tree(s) are at a desired size, the allergy producing tree(s) can be removed. This process can take three to ten years, but usually occurs between three and six years.

◼ Hiring a Professional

If you are not an outdoor person or just do not have a green thumb, then I suggest hiring a qualified landscape professional to design, rearrange and/or install your allergy-free landscape. A knowledgeable landscape professional should be licensed and insured. Professionals can range from a landscape design company to a nurserymen to a landscape architect. Simple tree and shrub removal can be accomplished by a professional tree trimmer or licensed certified arborist.

Once you have decided on a landscape professional, start looking through the allergy-free chapter and list plants that you would like designed into your landscape and communicate this to your landscape professional. Emphasize the use of allergy-free plants and the need to remove designated allergy producing plants. Your landscape professional should have a copy of this book. He or she will then design your landscape based on the information you provide. Several drafts may need to be drawn before you settle on a final plan. Once the final plans are approved and a price is agreed upon, the allergy-free landscape can begin and you can start to enjoy your immediate landscape environment.

◼ Repetition

The three places you most frequently occupy are your home, work, and surrounding community. The repeated use of allergy-free plants in these places will make an impact on reducing the severity and longevity of allergy symptoms. Replacing allergy producing plants with allergy-free plants will reduce the current levels of allergy provoking pollen in the air we breath. It will take time to reverse the trend and reduce the levels of pollen in the air. Today is the best day to start reducing your allergy symptoms. Start acting, start removing, start planting, then start enjoying.

◼ Alternate Steps in Reducing Pollen

There will be cases where allergy producing plants cannot be removed. These situations generally have to do with factors such as money constraints, timing, and environment. Don't panic, there are a few methods of reducing the output of pollen from allergy provoking plants.

Turf Grass:
The key to controlling turf grass pollen is keeping it mowed and edged on a weekly basis. Consistent and timely mowing of lawn grasses keeps

them from forming a flower spike which holds the pollen grains. This is especially true with common bermuda grass.

Keep common bermuda grass cut short, 1" to 2" tall. Bermuda grass tends to escape the intended lawn areas and spread into flower beds, gardens, bare areas, and concrete cracks. In these areas, common bermuda grass can be neglected or overlooked, thus allowing it time to grow a flower spike and produce pollen. Pull, hoe or spray all unwanted areas of bermuda grass. When spraying use an appropriate weed killer, preferably one with systemic qualities. Take care not to spray desired plants or you may kill them too. Some weed killers only kill grasses, but be careful, some landscape plants are actually a grass. Consult a landscape professional for more information and assistance.

A fairly inexpensive way to change bermuda grass into a fescue grass is to mow your lawn short (1" or shorter); then, spray the bermuda grass with a systemic weed and grass killer. Several days after spraying you can overseed the lawn area with fescue seed. Apply 1/4" of humus over the top and keep the seed moist for one to two weeks until the new seed germinates. This is a quick and successful way to reduce allergy symptoms caused by bermuda grass.

The only drawback is that the bermuda may come back in a few places. Even the best application of weed and grass killer can leave a few pieces of live grass. However, repeated spraying and overseeding can remedy the situation.

Shrubs and Trees:

If an allergy producing plant can't be removed then I suggest its size be reduced by pruning whenever possible. Most plants can be pruned properly without ruining their looks, health or structural integrity. One exception may be birch trees, especially in hotter climates, because they generally don't respond well to being pruned frequently. Some trees like mulberry, are pollarded (pruned) every year. This severely reduces the amount of pollen production. Consult a certified arborist (tree expert) for more information.

Spraying an allergy producing plant with water at the time the pollen is emerging from the plant is a good way to keep a lot of the pollen from becoming airborne. Repeated spraying will be needed during the plant's pollinating period. Some trees like sycamore, Chinese elm and ash shouldn't be sprayed with water, especially in the spring and early summer. They can get a fungal disorder called anthracnose which defoliates the tree. If this occurs you should consult a certified arborist.

Weeds:

Weeds can be a major source of allergy misery. They do not have to be. The key is the early and consistent killing of the emerging weed plants. Many people use a pre-emergent herbicide which kills most of the weed seeds in the ground as they start to germinate. Some use weed killers while others hoe or pull them. It is a constant battle, but one that must be fought.

The highest concentration of weeds in the cities comes from vacant or open lots, parks, ditches, rivers, ponds, lakes, and streams. Weeds in rural areas are concentrated along roadsides, farm ground, waste places, pastures, ditches, rivers, and streams, vacant or natural areas, and abandoned land. Community involvement is needed to severely reduce the weed population in the cities. Rural weed control involves the coordination and cooperation of county, state, and federal officials, as well as farmers, ranchers, and rural citizens.

▪ A Note About Schools

Allergies from plant pollen contributes to the absenteeism of thousands of our school children every year. The learning time lost from absenteeism and the reduced learning capacity of children from allergy symptoms while in school is astounding. Revenue lost from student absences cost school districts undeterminable amounts of money. Sports, band and scholastic activities are all effected by poor student participation and or absence. Inhalers, antihistamines and steroids are all too common words to our children.

Medications to lessen the reactions to allergies are a big help to those in need, but many still have some unwanted side effects. In some cases supplemental use of allergy medications turns into a co-dependency relationship. "Can we *reduce* school absenteeism and *increase* student health by removing allergy producing plants on our school grounds? It is worth a try. Our children's health is at stake."

▪ Prevention — the Best Medicine

To date, medicine treats the symptoms, but doesn't provide the cure. It is often said prevention is the best medicine. However, we tend to think, "prevention" as a limiting word like moderation, abstinence or avoidance. If we look at prevention as a medicine not as a phrase, we can then begin to see the possibilities and opportunities open to us. Prevent something from happening or reduce something from happening by preventing or limiting its contact with you. Removing allergy producing plants and planting allergy-free plants is a preventative measure to reduce your allergy severity and recurrence. This type of prevention is a liberating process, which allows for a more enjoyable activity.

Business Owners

The loss to employers from lost or unproductive man hours from allergy related causes, is in excess of 1 billion dollars annually. In many cases, the business landscape environment adds to this figure significantly. The cost to remove allergy producing plants and replace them with allergy-free plants at work could be recouped by higher employee attendance and productivity. Think back and remember how many times employees have been sick from allergies. Find out how many people in your employment have allergies. Locate all allergy producing plants at work and, if possible, your employee's homes. Decide the cost to remove and re-plant versus the lost money from employee down time. Amortize this over many years and you will find it will actually save you money. If possible, start an employer/employee incentive program where the business helps defer the cost of removing allergy producing plants from the employee's homes. This could be given in the form of a bonus. Check with a tax consultant for a way to deduct the expense from your business. People helping people. That's how ideas and plans succeed. It's a win-win situation.

Medical Institutions

Medical institutions like hospitals, doctor's offices, and convalescent facilities, should be sensitive to patients' allergy conditions. The creation of allergy-free zones on all medical property will help comfort and reduce patients' and their visitors' allergy symptoms. Going to or visiting a hospital is often an emotional and traumatic experience. Allergy susceptibility is often higher in times of emotional stress. Patients and visitors do not need the added exposure to allergy provoking plants during a visit to a hospital or medical facility. The creation of an allergy-free landscape on medical campuses is

a big plus for the doctors, nurses, and staff as well. Allergy symptoms like sneezing, are unsterile and can complicate some medical procedures or practices. Recognizing allergy producing plants as a disease-causing medical problem, will change the way we think and act about our outdoor environment.

Therapy Landscapes

There's been a lot of emphasis placed on the mental and physical effects a beautifully landscaped pavilion or courtyard can have on the healing of patients. Warm and inviting, these areas can be a haven for ill and recovering patients. However, for some patients these areas can be an illness waiting to happen. Sneezing and wheezing, especially after an abdominal surgery, can be very painful. Designers of therapy courtyards or landscapes must be fully aware of what plants are appropriate for these types of areas. Not only must allergy-free plants be incorporated, but also special consideration must be given to edible plants, plants that attract wanted or unwanted animals and insects, and avoiding poisonous plants. We have a need. The technology is here; we just have to use it.

Government Entities

City, county, state, and federal entities govern many of our outdoor landscape areas. This includes streets, parks, roads, freeways, and government buildings. All of these areas have landscaping associated with them. The unilateral adoption of planting allergy-free plants in our government-run areas would be a giant step forward in the battle against allergies. Policies should be adopted outlining the use of allergy-free plants in public areas. Hopefully, voluntary compliance will be enacted instead of mandatory laws.

Landscape Professionals

Landscape designers, installers, contractors, landscape architects, engineers, and architects can also make a big difference in reducing the allergy symptoms by specifying allergy-free plants in their landscape designs. The landscape professionals will need to educate themselves first, then the client about the benefits of having an allergy-free landscape. These professionals design a large portion of our city landscapes. It would be wonderful if they started designing "allergy-free."

◼ *Starting Point*

First, we need to start reducing allergy producing plants where we live. Second, where we work. And last, in our community. Many civic and plant-minded organizations already exist in most communities across the nation. Some of them may include garden clubs, beautification committees, street tree committees, government agencies, service clubs, business affiliates, and health clubs. Contact these and other organizations for help in forming and enacting guidelines to reduce the allergy producing plants in the community. Many people working individually and together, will make a difference in our communities.

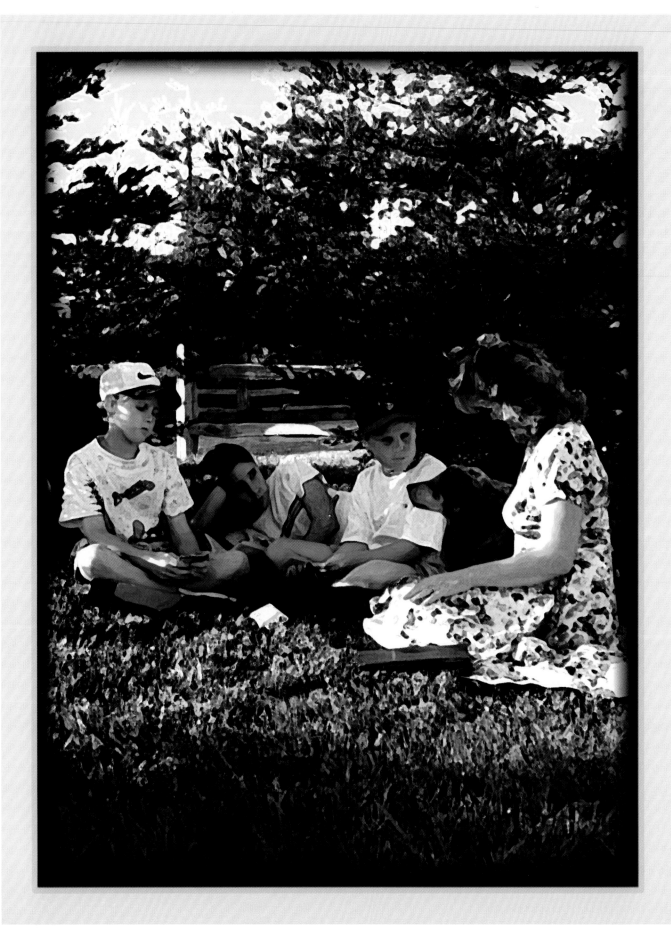

Chapter 5

Allergy-Free Plants and Low Pollen Producers

◤ *Definition*

A plant is said to be allergy-free or a low pollen producer if the pollen produced by the plant is significantly low in numbers or doesn't produce pollen, or if the physical properties of the pollen (sticky, heavy) make it nearly impossible for it to become or stay airborne. Once a person is exposed to the pollen of these plants their body does not react negatively, (causing allergy symptoms). Of course, there will always be exceptions to the rule. That is, because everyone is different in their genetic makeup there will always be some who can be allergic to an allergy-free or low pollen producing plant. However, the number of people in this category is very, very small.

◤ *Explanation of Format*

The purpose of this chapter is to identify the plants that are allergy-free or low pollen producers and explain how to use them in a landscape by uncovering their unique habits and characteristics in an easy to read and understandable format. The plants are listed in alphabetical order by the **Botanical Name** which is listed at the top of each page with the **Common Name** below it. You can use the index to look up any plant's common name if you are not familiar with its botanical name. A botanical name index is also included.

The type of information you will find for each allergy-free or low pollen producing plant is, the botanical name in alphabetical order with the common name below. Next is the **USDA Climate Zones** identifying the geographic areas where the plant can grow according to its cold temperature tolerance. The **Origin** of the plant is listed for informational purposes. The **Form** lists the size and shape of the plant. The **Description** explains the size, color, shape and general appearance of the foilage. The next four characteristics will help in the placement of each plant in the landscape. They are **Flower Color, Exposure, Water,** and **Growth Rate.** Individual **Char-**

acteristics are listed next. This will assist in understanding the regional requirements the plants may need or can tolerate. These would include drought, heat tolerances, special fertilizer needs, special pruning requirements, plants that are susceptible to insects and diseases, flower fragrances, odors, and much more.

Lastly, the general and specific **Uses** are listed. They include accent, border, understory, mass planting, screen, wind block, plants to use around pools, walkways, old fashion gardens, patios, shade tree, specimen, medicinal uses and much more.

The intent is for readers to use these allergy-free or low pollen producing plants instead of allergy producing plants in their landscapes at home, at the office and in their surrounding community and to have sufficient knowledge of plant characteristics so that intelligent planting choices can be made.

◤ *USDA Plant Hardiness Zone Map*

The USDA Zones map, located on the next page, indicates the approximate range of minimum temperatures for the United States. It is broken down into 11 zones with 1 being the coldest -50°F and 11 the warmest at 40°F. These zones are basic and do not indicate other climatic characteristics such as rainfall, maximum temperatures, humidity, and aridness. Use these zones as a guide. Further climatic information may be needed for your specific area.

USDA Plant Hardiness Zone Map

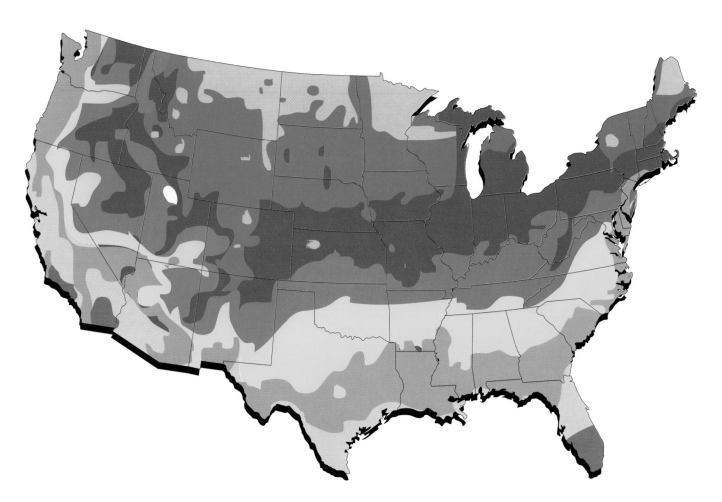

Range of Average Annual Minimum Temperature for each Zone

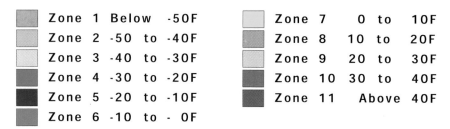

Zone 1	Below	-50F
Zone 2	-50 to	-40F
Zone 3	-40 to	-30F
Zone 4	-30 to	-20F
Zone 5	-20 to	-10F
Zone 6	-10 to	- 0F

Zone 7	0 to	10F
Zone 8	10 to	20F
Zone 9	20 to	30F
Zone 10	30 to	40F
Zone 11	Above	40F

BOTANICAL NAME: *Abelia grandiflora*
COMMON NAME: GLOSSY ABELIA
USDA ZONES: 6, 7, 8, 9, 10, 11
ORIGIN: Hybrid from China
FORM: Evergreen to partially deciduous broadleaf shrub, up to 8' tall by 5' wide
DESCRIPTION: Green to bronzy leaves, 1/2" to 1-1/2" long, attached to arching stems originating from the base
FLOWER COLOR: Light pink, blooms from summer to fall
EXPOSURE: Full sun to partial shade
WATER: Moderate
GROWTH RATE: Moderate to rapid
CHARACTERISTICS: Will not tolerate reflected heat, constant or high winds or salty soils. Selectively prune, do not shear. Prune before new growth appears in winter. Fertilize lightly in summer and fall.
USES: Use as a background or filler plant, erosion control, low screen, border, and divider. Will add color and texture to most landscapes. Mixes well with dark green foliage.

BOTANICAL NAME: *Abelia grandiflora 'Edward Goucher'*
COMMON NAME: EDWARD GOUCHER ABELIA
USDA ZONES: 6, 7, 8, 9, 10, 11
ORIGIN: Hybrid from China
FORM: Evergreen to partially deciduous broadleaf shrub, up to 5' tall by 3' wide
DESCRIPTION: Green to bronzy leaves, 1" to 1-1/2" long, attached to arching stems originating from the base, lacier than *Abelia grandiflora*
FLOWER COLOR: Medium pink, 3/4" long, blooms from summer to fall
EXPOSURE: Full sun to partial shade
WATER: Moderate
GROWTH RATE: Moderate to rapid
CHARACTERISTICS: Will not tolerate reflected heat, constant or high winds or salty soils. Selectively prune, do not shear. Prune before new growth appears in winter. Fertilize lightly in summer and fall.
USES: Use as a background or filler plant, erosion control, low screen, border, and divider. Will add color and texture to most landscapes. Mixes well with dark green foliage.

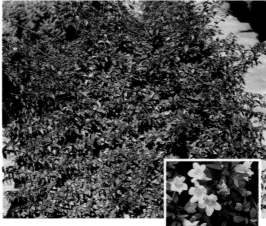

BOTANICAL NAME: *Aloysia triphylla*
COMMON NAME: LEMON VERBENA
USDA ZONES: 8, 9, 10, 11
ORIGIN: South America
FORM: Deciduous to partially evergreen broadleaf shrub, up to 6' tall
DESCRIPTION: Green leaves, 3" long, narrow in shape, in whorls of 2 to 4
FLOWER COLOR: Whitish to lilac, tiny, blooms in summer
EXPOSURE: Full sun
WATER: Moderate, well-drained soil
GROWTH RATE: Moderate
CHARACTERISTICS: Lemon-scented leaves. Can get leggy. Prune back to invigorate new growth.
USES: Leaves used in cold drinks, and apple jelly.

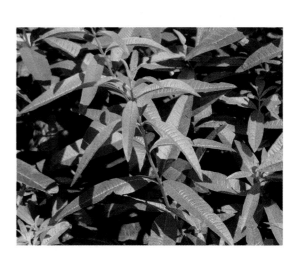

BOTANICAL NAME: *Arctostaphylos densiflora*
COMMON NAME: SONOMA MANZANITA
USDA ZONES: 8
ORIGIN: Sonoma County in California
FORM: Woody evergreen broadleaf shrub, 4' to 6' tall
DESCRIPTION: Light to dark green glossy leaves, 1-1/4" long
FLOWER COLOR: Rosy-pink, 1/4" wide, bell-shaped, blooms in spring
EXPOSURE: Full sun to partial shade
WATER: Moderate until established, then once a month during dry seasons
GROWTH RATE: Moderate
CHARACTERISTICS: Best in loose, well-drained soils. Does well in natural settings with other low water requiring plants. Aphids and green scale are a problem. Mounding or creeping growth habit.
USES: Native setting, bank cover, hillside, slope, ground cover, near rocks, and understory.

BOTANICAL NAME: *Arctostaphylos hookeri*
COMMON NAME: HOOKER MANZANITA
USDA ZONES: 2, 3, 4, 5, 6, 7, 8
ORIGIN: California north to Alaska
FORM: Woody evergreen broadleaf shrub, up to 6' tall by 6' wide
DESCRIPTION: Bright green glossy leaves, about 3/4" long, oval in shape
FLOWER COLOR: Pinkish, 1/4" wide, bell-shaped, blooms from late winter to early spring
EXPOSURE: Full sun to partial shade
WATER: Moderate until established, then once a month during dry seasons
GROWTH RATE: Moderate
CHARACTERISTICS: Tolerates heat and drought once established. Does well in alkaline soils, coastal conditions, and inland climates. Aphids can be a problem. Constant overhead irrigation can lead to fungal problems which often kills manzanita. Pruning is seldom needed. Tip pinch occasionally to keep plant full. Bark is a deep red.
USES: Native setting, bank cover, hillside, areas of little irrigation, near rocks, and tall ground cover.

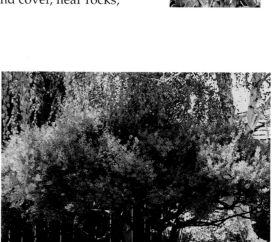

BOTANICAL NAME: *Arctostaphylos uva-ursi*
COMMON NAME: CREEPING MANZANITA
USDA ZONES: 2, 3, 4, 5, 6, 7, 8
ORIGIN: San Mateo County in California north to Alaska
FORM: Woody evergreen low-growing broadleaf shrub or ground cover, up to 1' tall
DESCRIPTION: Bright green glossy leaves, turning reddish in winter, leathery texture, 1" long
FLOWER COLOR: Whitish-pink, 1/4" wide, bell-shaped, blooms in early spring
EXPOSURE: Full sun to partial shade
WATER: Moderate, low to infrequent thereafter
GROWTH RATE: Slow at first, moderate when established
CHARACTERISTICS: Prostrate growth habit. Branches root when in contact with soil. Seasonal red berries.
USES: Native setting, ground cover, steep bank, hillside, cascading on wall, understory, and near rocks.

BOTANICAL NAME: *Asparagus densiflorus 'Myers'*
COMMON NAME: **ASPARAGUS FERN**
USDA ZONES: 9, 10, house plant
ORIGIN: Europe
FORM: Semi-herbaceous evergreen shrub
DESCRIPTION: Medium to light green cladodes, 1/4" long,
                   amassed on long plumes, up to 2' tall
FLOWER COLOR: White, small
EXPOSURE: Partial shade best
WATER: Moderate
GROWTH RATE: Moderate to fast
CHARACTERISTICS: Tolerates drought conditions due to
                   water-holding tubers within the roots.
                   Wear gloves when handling this plant to
                   avoid the tiny spines on the stems. Fertilize
                   monthly in containers.
USES: Mostly used as a house plant. Patio, planter, shady ground cover, and flower arrangement
                   (foliage).

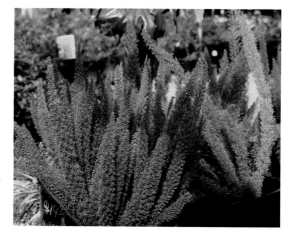

BOTANICAL NAME: *Asparagus densiflorus 'Sprengeri'*
COMMON NAME: **SPRENGER ASPARAGUS**
USDA ZONES: 9, 10, house plant
ORIGIN: Europe
FORM: Semi-herbaceous evergreen vining shrub
DESCRIPTION: Medium to light green glossy cladodes,
                   3/4" to 1" long, needle-like in shape
FLOWER COLOR: Inconspicuous
EXPOSURE: Full sun to partial shade
WATER: Moderate
GROWTH RATE: Moderate to fast
CHARACTERISTICS: Tolerates drought conditions due to water-
                   holding tubers within the root system. Wear
                   gloves to avoid touching the tiny spines on
                   the stems. Fertilize monthly in containers.
USES: Mostly a house plant or used as a container plant on patio, ground cover,
                   trellis, and shady ground cover.

BOTANICAL NAME: *Aspidistra elatior*
COMMON NAME: **CAST-IRON PLANT**
USDA ZONES: 8, house plant, anywhere
ORIGIN: Himalayas, Taiwan, China, Japan
FORM: Semi-herbaceous evergreen perennial
                   broadleaf shrub
DESCRIPTION: Green glossy leaves, semi-rough texture,
                   1' to 2-1/2' long by 3" to 4" wide, blade-like
                   in shape, flat, arching, parallel veins
FLOWER COLOR: Inconspicuous
EXPOSURE: Filtered to deep shade
WATER: Moderate
GROWTH RATE: Moderate
CHARACTERISTICS: Tolerates neglect and poor growing
                   conditions well, but for best results fertilize

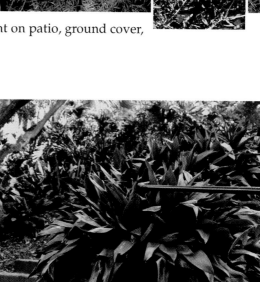

occasionally and apply moderate water. Excellent shade plant. Syringe foliage to keep dust
off. Foliage will burn in full sun.
USES: Most any shady situation indoor or out. Shaded patio, entryway, walkway, understory,
                   and flower arrangement.

BOTANICAL NAME: *Aucuba japonica*
COMMON NAME: **JAPANESE AUCUBA**
USDA ZONES: 7, 8
ORIGIN: Japan
FORM: Woody evergreen broadleaf shrub, 6' to 10' tall
DESCRIPTION: Dark green glossy leaves, 3" to 8" long by 1-1/2" to 3" wide, oblong in shape, serrate margins on upper half
FLOWER COLOR: Purple, inconspicuous
EXPOSURE: Full to partial shade
WATER: Moderate, drought tolerant once established
GROWTH RATE: Moderate
CHARACTERISTICS: Leaves will burn if planted in full sun. Scale, mealybugs, aphids, and snails can be a problem. Prune occasionally to keep compact. Variegated varieties available.
USES: Shady conditions, accent, understory, container, and tropical setting. Good in conjunction with ferns, hydrangeas, and azaleas.

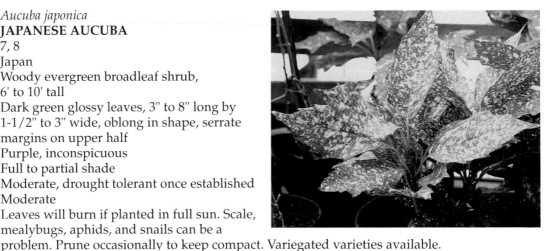

BOTANICAL NAME: *Azalea spp.*
COMMON NAME: **AZALEA**
USDA ZONES: 3, 4, 5, 6, 7, 8, 9
ORIGIN: China
FORM: Woody mostly evergreen broadleaf shrub, 1' to 6' tall
DESCRIPTION: Light to dark green leaves, 1/2" to 1" long, oval to oblong in shape
FLOWER COLOR: White, pink, red, lavender, salmon, orange, magenta, bi-colors, 2" to 4" wide, funnel-shaped, blooms in spring
EXPOSURE: Full sun to partial shade
WATER: Moderate and moist
GROWTH RATE: Moderate
CHARACTERISTICS: Keep soil pH on the acidic side with good drainage. Pinch tips after flowering to keep bushy. Fertilize lightly after flowering and a few times during summer. Grows best in western shade.
USES: Spring color, accent, container, house plant, mass planting, and understory especially in woodsy or oriental-type setting. Very versatile, and widely used plant.

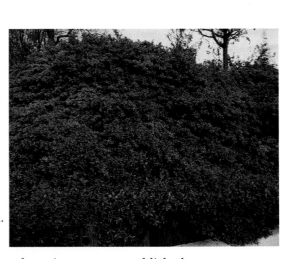

BOTANICAL NAME: *Baccharis pilularis*
COMMON NAME: **COYOTE BRUSH**
USDA ZONES: 8
ORIGIN: California coastal hills
FORM: Woody evergreen mounding broadleaf shrub, up to 2' tall by 6' wide
DESCRIPTION: Bright green leaves, 1/2" to 1" long, simple, serrate margins
FLOWER COLOR: Inconspicuous
EXPOSURE: Full sun
WATER: Moderate, low thereafter
GROWTH RATE: Moderate to fast
CHARACTERISTICS: Prune in late winter just before spring growth. Plant on 2' to 3' centers if mass planting. Very little or no fertilizer is needed. Good low maintenance shrub. Fire retardant and drought resistant once established.
USES: Hillside, rock garden, native planting, drier or infrequently irrigated areas, and ground cover.

BOTANICAL NAME: *Berberis thunbergii*
COMMON NAME: GREEN BARBERRY
USDA ZONES: 4, 5, 6, 7, 8, 9
ORIGIN: Japan
FORM: Woody upright deciduous broadleaf shrub, up to 4' tall by 6' wide
DESCRIPTION: Dark green leaves, lighter green underneath, 1/2" long by 1-1/2" wide
FLOWER COLOR: Yellow, tiny, blooms in spring
EXPOSURE: Full sun
WATER: Moderate, keep moist
GROWTH RATE: Moderate
CHARACTERISTICS: Good fall color. Spines on branches, red berries in the fall and winter. Transplants easily. Best if kept informal. Tip pinch to keep compact. Tolerates heat, wind, dust, smoke, short durations of drought.
USES: Good physical barrier, hedge, fall color (yellow, orange, red), accent, and oriental setting. Good against light green background such as xylosma, boxwood, and understory.

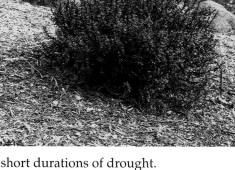

BOTANICAL NAME: *Berberis thunbergii 'Atropurpurea'*
COMMON NAME: RED BARBERRY
USDA ZONES: 4, 5, 6, 7, 8, 9
ORIGIN: Japan
FORM: Woody upright deciduous broadleaf shrub, up to 4' tall by 6' wide
DESCRIPTION: Bronzy-red leaves, light green underneath, 1/2" to 1-1/2" long
FLOWER COLOR: Yellow, tiny, blooms in spring
EXPOSURE: Full sun
WATER: Moderate, keep moist
GROWTH RATE: Moderate
CHARACTERISTICS: Good fall color. Spines on branches, red berries in fall and winter. Transplants easily. Best if kept informal. Tip pinch to keep compact. Tolerates heat, wind, dust, smoke, short durations of drought.
USES: Good physical barrier, hedge, fall color (yellow, orange, red), accent, and oriental setting. Good against light green background such as xylosma, boxwood, and understory plant.

BOTANICAL NAME: *Bougainvillea spectabilis*
COMMON NAME: BOUGAINVILLEA
USDA ZONE: 9, 10
ORIGIN: Brazil
FORM: Woody evergreen sprawling broadleaf vine
DESCRIPTION: Dark green leaves, velvety texture, 2" to 4" long, oval in shape
FLOWER COLOR: Purple, pink, salmon, red, gold, white, 1" to 2" long, blooms from late spring to early fall
EXPOSURE: Full sun
WATER: Moderate, keep moist
GROWTH RATE: Fast
CHARACTERISTICS: Hard to transplant. Best to cut container and keep rootball intact while planting. Plant can die from disrupting the rootball during planting. Support is needed to stay erect. Fertilize lightly once or twice per year. Plant after frost season in spring for best results. Thorns on stems.
USES: Accent, flower color, trellis, barrier, entryway, fence, and chimney cover (keep away from top).

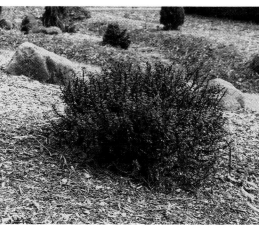
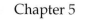

BOTANICAL NAME: *Brunfelsia calycina 'Floribunda'*
COMMON NAME: **YESTERDAY-TODAY-TOMORROW**
USDA ZONES: 8, 9
ORIGIN: Tropic America
FORM: Woody upright evergreen broadleaf shrub, up to 10' tall
DESCRIPTION: Dark green leaves, lighter green underneath, 3" to 4" long, oval in shape
FLOWER COLOR: First purple, then lavender, turning to white, 2" wide, blooms from spring to early summer
EXPOSURE: Partial to half shade best
WATER: Moderate, keep moist
GROWTH RATE: Moderate
CHARACTERISTICS: Needs extra attention. Provide a well amended acidic soil. Fertilize throughout growing and flowering seasons. Add iron if chlorotic symptoms appear. Prune to shape and invigorate. Looses most of its leaves in winter for a short period.
USES: Accent, flower color, container, patio, entryway, shaded area, and understory.

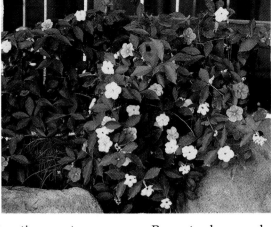

BOTANICAL NAME: *Buddleia alternifolia*
COMMON NAME: **FOUNTAIN BUTTERFLY BUSH, ALTERNATE-LEAF BUDDLEIA**
USDA ZONES: 5, 6, 7, 8, 9
ORIGIN: Tropic and subtropic South and North America, Africa, Asia
FORM: Woody deciduous broadleaf shrub or small tree, up to 12' tall
DESCRIPTION: Dark green dull leaves, lighter pubescent underneath, 1" to 4" long by 3/4" wide
FLOWER COLOR: Purple, mildly fragrant, blooms in spring
EXPOSURE: Full sun to light shade
WATER: Moderate
GROWTH RATE: Moderate
CHARACTERISTICS: Blooms on previous season's growth so prune only after blooming period to insure massive blooms for next year. Tolerates many types of soil. Branches are long and arching.
USES: Seasonal accent, border, specimen, flower color, and small tree.

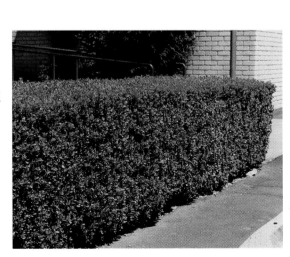

BOTANICAL NAME: *Buxus microphylla 'Japonica'*
COMMON NAME: **JAPANESE BOXWOOD**
USDA ZONES: 5, 6, 7, 8, 9
ORIGIN: Japan
FORM: Woody evergreen broadleaf shrub, 4' to 6' tall
DESCRIPTION: Medium green leaves, turning bronzy-red in winter, 1/3" to 1" long, oval in shape
FLOWER COLOR: Inconspicuous
EXPOSURE: Full sun to light shade
WATER: Moderate
GROWTH RATE: Slow to moderate
CHARACTERISTICS: A good hardy plant tolerant of many conditions including dry heat, alkaline soils and hot sun. Pest problems include spider mites, nematodes, and scale. Takes pruning well.
USES: Formal hedge, barrier, container, and low screen.

BOTANICAL NAME: *Caesalpinia gilliesii*
COMMON NAME: **BIRD OF PARADISE**
USDA ZONES: 9
ORIGIN: Argentina, Uruguay
FORM: Woody evergreen (deciduous in cold winter areas) upright broadleaf shrub or small tree, up to 10' tall
DESCRIPTION: Green leaves, 1" long, finely cut margins covered with a thin layer of film
FLOWER COLOR: Yellow, small, 4" to 5" red stamens, blooms all summer
EXPOSURE: Full sun
WATER: Infrequent and deep
GROWTH RATE: Fast
CHARACTERISTICS: Tough hardy plant. Drops all of its leaves in areas where winters are cold. Flowers all summer long. Good plant to attract hummingbirds.
USES: Summer accent, rock gardens, small tree, and border.

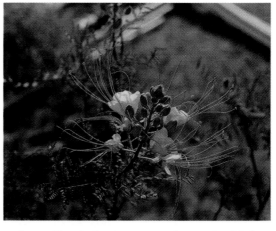

BOTANICAL NAME: *Calycanthus occidentalis*
COMMON NAME: **WESTERN SPICE BUSH**
USDA ZONES: 4, 5, 6, 7, 8, 9
ORIGIN: California coast and Sierra Nevada foothills
FORM: Woody deciduous broadleaf shrub or small tree, 4' to 12' tall
DESCRIPTION: Bright green leaves, turning yellow in fall, light pubescence underneath, 2" to 8" long by 1" to 2" wide, oblong in shape
FLOWER COLOR: Purplish-red brown, 2" wide, lily-like, fragrant, blooms in summer
EXPOSURE: Full sun to partial shade
WATER: Moderate
GROWTH RATE: Moderate
CHARACTERISTICS: Flowers and leaves are fragrant when crushed. Regenerate growth by pruning out 1/3 of existing growth to the ground.
USES: Specimen, riparian setting, moist slope, color, border, and fragrance.

BOTANICAL NAME: *Camellia japonica*
COMMON NAME: **JAPANESE CAMELLIA**
USDA ZONES: 7, 8, 9, 10
ORIGIN: Asia
FORM: Woody evergreen broadleaf shrub, 6' to 20' tall
DESCRIPTION: Dark green glossy leaves, leathery texture, 3-1/2" long by 1-1/2" wide, oval in shape, pointed at the tip
FLOWER COLOR: White, pink, red, single, double, 2-1/2" to 5" wide, blooms in spring
EXPOSURE: Partial afternoon shade best
WATER: Moderate, keep moist
GROWTH RATE: Slow to moderate
CHARACTERISTICS: Sensitive to hard frost. Prune out spent flowers and discard in trash or risk of fungal disorders increase. Can get leaf spot, and scale. Keep soil pH on the acidic side. Many colors are available, check your local nursery.
USES: Shady area, understory, oriental setting, planter, container, patio, and bonsai.

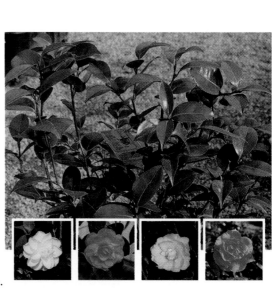

BOTANICAL NAME: *Camellia sasanqua*
COMMON NAME: **SASANQUA CAMELLIA**
USDA ZONES: 7, 8, 9
ORIGIN: Asia
FORM: Woody evergreen broadleaf shrub, generally 6' to 12' tall, varies within varieties
DESCRIPTION: Dark green glossy leaves, leathery texture, 2-1/2" long by 1-1/2" wide, oval in shape, thick, pointed at the tip
FLOWER COLOR: White, pink, red, single, double, 2" to 5" wide, blooms in fall
EXPOSURE: Afternoon shade best
WATER: Moderate, keep moist
GROWTH RATE: Slow to moderate
CHARACTERISTICS: Sensitive to hard frost. Flowers appear in the fall. Prune out spent flowers and discard in trash or risk of fungal disorders increase. Can get Phytophora cinnamoni root rot, petal blight, leaf spot, and scale. Keep soil pH acidic. Many colors are available. Petals can be damaged by frost and rain.
USES: Shady area, understory, oriental setting, planter, container, patio, bonsai, and fall accent.

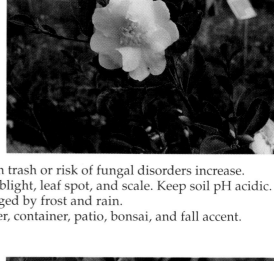

BOTANICAL NAME: *Campsis grandiflora (Bignonia chinensis)*
COMMON NAME: **TRUMPET VINE**
USDA ZONES: 8
ORIGIN: China
FORM: Woody deciduous broadleaf vine
DESCRIPTION: Medium green leaves, 2-1/2" long, compound with 9 to 11 leaflets
FLOWER COLOR: Scarlet, 2" to 3" wide, blooms in summer
EXPOSURE: Full sun
WATER: Moderate
GROWTH RATE: Fast
CHARACTERISTICS: Will cling to almost anything including wood, brick, and concrete. Root system invasive and reproduced by suckering roots (rhizomes). Hard to get rid of once established. Best planted where roots are confined to an area such as containers. Needs support. Train into a shrub by pruning branches very short.
USES: Flowering vine, ground cover, big shrub, flowering hedge, container, screen, and espalier.

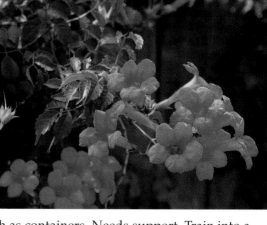

BOTANICAL NAME: *Carissa grandiflora*
COMMON NAME: **NATAL PLUM**
USDA ZONES: 9
ORIGIN: South Africa
FORM: Woody evergreen mounding broadleaf shrub, up to 7' tall
DESCRIPTION: Dark green leaves, leathery texture, 3" long, oval in shape, spines on branches and ends of each twig
FLOWER COLOR: White, 2" wide, fragrant, blooms lightly all year
EXPOSURE: Full sun best for flowering, partial shade otherwise
WATER: Moderate
GROWTH RATE: Fast
CHARACTERISTICS: Tolerates ocean winds and salt spray. Flowers are fragrant, resembling the smell of jasmine. The sharp spines if contacted, can cause considerable pain or injury.
USES: Physical barrier, informal or prune closely for formal hedge, and container.

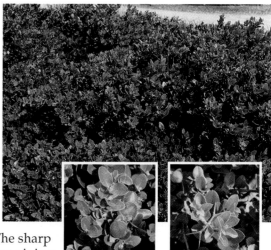
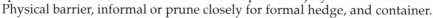

■ BOTANICAL NAME: *Carpenteria californica*
COMMON NAME: BUSH ANEMONE
USDA ZONES: 7
ORIGIN: California Sierra Nevada foothills and along
                  the Kings and San Joaquin rivers
FORM: Woody evergreen broadleaf shrub, 3' to 6' tall
DESCRIPTION: Dark green leaves, whitish pubescence
                  underneath, 4-1/2" long by 1" wide, oblong
                  in shape, thick, new bark turns purplish and
                  peels off with age
FLOWER COLOR: White, 1-1/2" to 3" wide, in clusters, mildly
                  fragrant, blooms from spring to summer
EXPOSURE: Partial shade best, full sun okay
WATER: Moderate
GROWTH RATE: Slow
CHARACTERISTICS: Resistant to oak root fungus. Attracts aphids. Prune out dead wood anytime. Prune live
                  wood after flowering to shape and promote next year's flowers.
USES: Native planting, specimen, and understory. Mixes with redbud and manzanita.

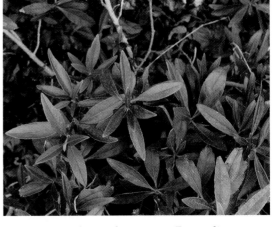

■ BOTANICAL NAME: *Chaenomeles speciosa*
COMMON NAME: FLOWERING QUINCE
USDA ZONES: 5, 6, 7, 8
ORIGIN: East Asia
FORM: Woody deciduous broadleaf shrub, 2' to 10' tall
DESCRIPTION: Medium green glossy leaves, small, young
                  foliage is dashed with red
FLOWER COLOR: Red-orange, pink, white-coral, purple-white,
                  salmon, 1-1/2" to 2-1/2" wide, blooms from
                  winter to late winter
EXPOSURE: Full sun
WATER: Moderate
GROWTH RATE: Moderate
CHARACTERISTICS: Picturesque but variable growth habit
                  especially in winter when branches are bare.
                  Very tough and durable plant. Tolerant of many types of soils (except alkaline), and
                  temperatures. One of the first plants to flower in late winter, early spring. Flower bud will
                  open indoors if cut after the new year. Thorns on attractive branches.
USES: Winter color, winter cut flower, physical barrier, accent, and oriental setting.

■ BOTANICAL NAME: *Cistus X hybridus*
COMMON NAME: WHITE ROCKROSE
USDA ZONES: 6, 7, 8
ORIGIN: Mediterranean area
FORM: Woody evergreen mounding broadleaf
                  shrub, up to 5' tall
DESCRIPTION: Pale to gray-green leaves, wrinkly texture,
                  2" long, oval in shape
FLOWER COLOR: White with yellow center, 1-1/2" wide, mildly
                  fragrant, blooms from spring to early summer
EXPOSURE: Full sun
WATER: Moderate, low once established
GROWTH RATE: Moderate to fast
CHARACTERISTICS: Established plants are drought tolerant and
                  can develop root rot if over watered. Once or
                  twice during summer months is sufficient. Likes well-drained soils on the acidic side.
USES: Native planting, desert situation, near rocks, erosion control, and ground cover.

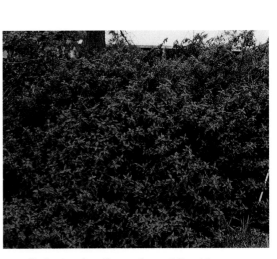

BOTANICAL NAME: *Cistus X purpureus*
COMMON NAME: **ORCHID ROCKROSE**
USDA ZONES: 6, 7, 8
ORIGIN: Mediterranean area
FORM: Woody evergreen mounding broadleaf shrub, up to 4' tall
DESCRIPTION: Pale to gray-green leaves, wrinkly texture, 1" to 2" long by 1/2" wide, narrow in shape
FLOWER COLOR: Reddish-purple with a red spot at the base, 3" wide, yellow stamens, blooms from spring to early summer
EXPOSURE: Full sun
WATER: Moderate, low once established
GROWTH RATE: Moderate to fast
CHARACTERISTICS: Established plants are drought tolerant and can develop root rot if over watered. Water once or twice during summer months is sufficient. Likes well-drained soils on the acidic side. Pinch tips to keep compact. Fire resistant.
USES: Native setting, areas of little or infrequent irrigation, desert situation, near rocks, erosion control, mass planting, tall ground cover, bank stabilizer, and roadway.

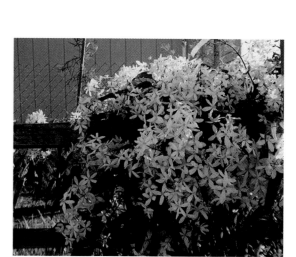

BOTANICAL NAME: *Clematis armandii*
COMMON NAME: **EVERGREEN CLEMATIS**
USDA ZONES: 4, 5, 6, 7, 8, 9
ORIGIN: China
FORM: Woody evergreen broadleaf vine, up to 20' long
DESCRIPTION: Dark green leaves, 3" to 5" long, compound with 3 leaflets, drooping appearance
FLOWER COLOR: Bright white, pink, 2-1/2" wide, in clusters, aromatic, blooms in early spring
EXPOSURE: Full sun, shade roots
WATER: Moderate
GROWTH RATE: Fast
CHARACTERISTICS: Leaves burn in salty soils. Slow growth until established. Prune after flowering to prevent buildup of dead inside branches and leaves. Must keep root system cool. Cover with at least 2" of mulch. Clematis does best if grown in an upward fashion (trellis). Flowers are aromatic.
USES: Trellis, fence cover, cut flower, railing, screen, arbor, and chimney (keep away from top).

BOTANICAL NAME: *Cocculus laurifolius*
COMMON NAME: **LAUREL-LEAF-SNAILSEED**
USDA ZONES: 8, 9, 10
ORIGIN: Himalayas
FORM: Woody evergreen broadleaf shrub or small tree, up to 25' tall
DESCRIPTION: Green glossy leaves, 6" long, simple, oblong in shape, pointed at the tip, 3 distinct veins running the entire length
FLOWER COLOR: Inconspicuous
EXPOSURE: Full sun to dense shade
WATER: Moderate, keep moist
GROWTH RATE: Moderate to fast once established
CHARACTERISTICS: Prune ends of branches to keep in shrub form or selectively thin out and stake to train into a multi-trunk tree. Tolerant of many soils. Very susceptible to cottony cushion scale.
USES: Understory, small umbrella-like shade tree, informal hedge, topiary, and background.

BOTANICAL NAME: *Cotoneaster dammeri*
COMMON NAME: **BEARBERRY COTONEASTER**
USDA ZONES: 5, 6, 7, 8
ORIGIN: West China
FORM: Woody evergreen sprawling broadleaf shrub, up to 10' long by 3" to 6" tall
DESCRIPTION: Bright green leaves, whitish underneath, 1" long, oval in shape, notched at the tip
FLOWER COLOR: Inconspicuous flowers, matures into red fruit
EXPOSURE: Full sun to partial shade
WATER: Moderate
GROWTH RATE: Fast
CHARACTERISTICS: Do not shear but selectively prune to shape. Give plenty of room to grow. Mass plantings should be spaced from 5' to 6' on center. Branches in contact with the ground will grow roots. Low growing. Susceptable to fireblight.
USES: Ground cover, near rocks, mass planting, bank cover, and winter color (berries).

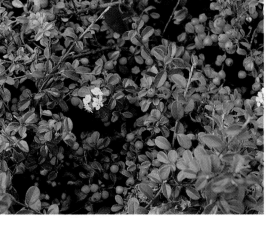

BOTANICAL NAME: *Cycas revoluta*
COMMON NAME: **SAGO**
USDA ZONES: 8
ORIGIN: Japan
FORM: Semi-woody evergreen shrub, up to 10' tall
DESCRIPTION: Green leaves, 2' to 3' long by 4" to 6" wide, looks like a cross between a fern and a palm, compound with numerous leaflets, very stiff, pointed at the tip, can poke if brushed against
FLOWER COLOR: Inconspicuous
EXPOSURE: Full sun, partial shade in hot climates
WATER: Moderate
GROWTH RATE: Very slow
CHARACTERISTICS: A very tough plant. Transplants easily although leaves may fall-off. They will sprout new leaves in time. Leaves grow in a whorl from the tip of the trunk (like a palm). Scale can be a problem, and leaf spot in areas of high humidity.
USES: Tropical or oriental effect, entryway, walkway, container, patio, indoor near high-light, gift, understory, accent, and arrangement (foliage).

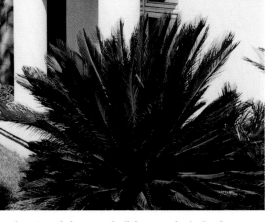

BOTANICAL NAME: *Cytisus racemosus (Genista racemosa)*
COMMON NAME: **EASTER BROOM**
USDA ZONES: 6, 7, 8
ORIGIN: Canary Island near Spain
FORM: Woody evergreen multi-stem broadleaf shrub, 3' to 8' tall
DESCRIPTION: Bright green leaves, 1/2" long, round in shape, some leaves have pubescence
FLOWER COLOR: Yellow spikes, 6" long by 3/4" wide, fragrant, blooms in late spring
EXPOSURE: Full sun
WATER: Moderate
GROWTH RATE: Fast
CHARACTERISTICS: Tolerates drought, wind, coastal conditions, rocky infertile soils, reseeds easily. Prune after blooming period.
USES: Screen, hedge, cut flower, areas of infrequent irrigation, good with western natives, accent, background, and rock garden.

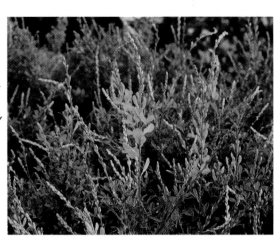

■ BOTANICAL NAME: *Datura (Brugmansia) suaveolens*
COMMON NAME: **ANGEL'S TRUMPET**
USDA ZONES: 9, 10, can be grown in pots
ORIGIN: Brazil
FORM: Woody evergreen broadleaf shrub, up to 15' tall
DESCRIPTION: Green dull leaves, 10" to 12" long, oval to lanceolate in shape
FLOWER COLOR: White flowers, green veins, 10" long, blooms in summer and fall
EXPOSURE: Full sun to half shade
WATER: Moderate, high during flowering
GROWTH RATE: Fast
CHARACTERISTICS: Unattractive when damaged by frost so cut back stems to 1 or 2 buds. Can be grown indoors. Flowers hang downward. Flowers and seeds are poisonous.
USES: Specimen, accent, color, rock garden, and background.

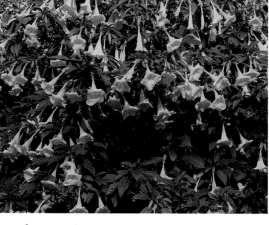

■ BOTANICAL NAME: *Diosma (Coleonema) pulchrum*
COMMON NAME: **BREATH OF HEAVEN**
USDA ZONES: 8, 9, 10
ORIGIN: South Africa
FORM: Woody evergreen broadleaf shrub, up to 5' tall
DESCRIPTION: Green leaves, heather-like texture, 1/4" long, narrow in shape, delicate, attached to slender branches
FLOWER COLOR: Pink, blooms from winter to spring
EXPOSURE: Full sun best, partial shade okay
WATER: Moderate, don't over water
GROWTH RATE: Moderate
CHARACTERISTICS: Provide good drainage. Plant parts are fragrant when crushed. Prune after flowering period. Shear to keep compact or thin out to promote upward growth.
USES: Near walkway, where foliage can be brushed up against to release fragrance, hillside, bank cover, and near building to soften their appearance.

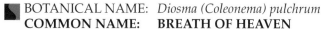

■ BOTANICAL NAME: *Ensete ventricosum (Musa ensete)*
COMMON NAME: **ABYSSINIAN BANANA**
USDA ZONES: 8, 9, 10, 11, indoors anywhere
ORIGIN: Ethiopia, Africa
FORM: Evergreen (palm like perennial shrub), 6' to 20' tall
DESCRIPTION: Green leaves, 10' to 20' long by 2' to 4' wide, distinctive midrib
FLOWER COLOR: Inconspicuous, blooms from spring to summer
EXPOSURE: Full sun to part shade
WATER: Moderate to high
GROWTH RATE: Fast
CHARACTERISTICS: Protect from the wind. Plant will die to the ground after flowering, however, it takes 2 to 5 years before plant will flower. Start new shoots from roots if desired.
USES: Indoor where there is room, near pool or other bodies of water, and tropical setting.

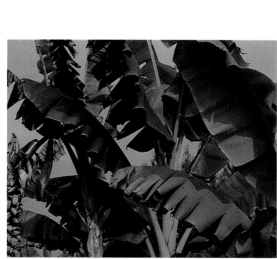

BOTANICAL NAME: *Erica spp.*
COMMON NAME: **HEATHER**
USDA ZONES: 8, 9
ORIGIN: South Africa
FORM: Woody evergreen broadleaf shrub, up to 6' tall
DESCRIPTION: Dark green leaves, whitish underneath, size varies, needle-like in shape
FLOWER COLOR: Pink, purple, 1/8" long, urn-shaped, blooms in late fall
EXPOSURE: Full sun on coast, partial shade inland
WATER: Moderate, keep moist
GROWTH RATE: Moderate

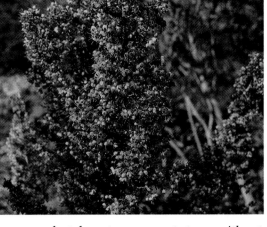

CHARACTERISTICS: Keep moist but not soggy. Absolutely not drought tolerant. Attracts bees. Provide good drainage and stay away from heavy clay soils and alkaline soils. Prune after blooms are gone but do not prune past stems without leaves or the stem will usually die back.
USES: Screen, excellent winter color, container plant, cut foliage, mass planting, rock garden. Goes well with azaleas, lily of the valley, and huckleberry.

BOTANICAL NAME: *Escallonia rubra*
COMMON NAME: **RED ESCALLONIA**
USDA ZONES: 7, 8, 9, 10
ORIGIN: South America, Chile, Argentina
FORM: Woody evergreen broadleaf shrub, 6' to 15' tall
DESCRIPTION: Dark green glossy leaves, smooth texture, up to 3" long, finely serrate margins, attached alternately to the stem
FLOWER COLOR: Red-crimson, 1" to 3" wide, in clusters, blooms from summer to fall
EXPOSURE: Full sun to partial shade
WATER: Moderate
GROWTH RATE: Fast

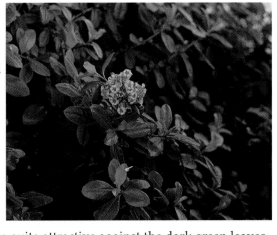

CHARACTERISTICS: Avoid heavy pruning or water sprouts will appear (prune only 25 to 33 percent of the shrub). Pinch tips to keep compact. Flowers are quite attractive against the dark green leaves.
USES: Background shrub, large screen, color, contrast with lighter colored shrubbery, and hedge.

BOTANICAL NAME: *Euryops pectinatus*
COMMON NAME: **GOLDEN SHRUB DAISY**
USDA ZONES: 8, 9, 10
ORIGIN: South Africa
FORM: Woody evergreen broadleaf shrub, up to 6' tall
DESCRIPTION: Medium to dark green leaves, 1" to 4" long, finely divided almost to the midrib
FLOWER COLOR: Yellow, 2" to 3" wide, daisy-like, on long slender flower stocks, blooms from late winter to fall of next year
EXPOSURE: Full sun best, partial shade okay
WATER: Moderate
GROWTH RATE: Moderate to fast in full sun

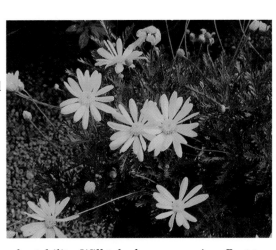

CHARACTERISTICS: Good staple or filler shrub with long blooming periods. Somewhat over used in California because of its flower color and wide adaptability. Will take heavy pruning. Best to prune in June. Perpetuate the flowering time by removing spent flowers.
USES: Color, accent, areas of high visibility where long lasting color is needed, border, and filler.

BOTANICAL NAME: *Fatsia japonica*
COMMON NAME: **JAPANESE ARALIA**
USDA ZONES: 7
ORIGIN: Japan
FORM: Woody evergreen upright broadleaf shrub, 5' to 8' tall
DESCRIPTION: Dark green leaves, 8" long, simple, lobed in shape (palm-like), attached to 12" to 16" semi-thick stalks
FLOWER COLOR: White, 10" long, in round clusters, foul smelling, not very showy, blooms in fall
EXPOSURE: Shade to partial shade best, will take full sun in milder areas
WATER: Moderate and moist
GROWTH RATE: Moderate
CHARACTERISTICS: Spray foliage to clean and reduce insects. Susceptible to aphids and scale. The flowers attract bees and flies. It's suggested to remove flower stalks before they open to eliminate problems and to keep stalks from branching.
USES: Container, patio, understory, tropical setting, and walkway. Looks good under night lighting.

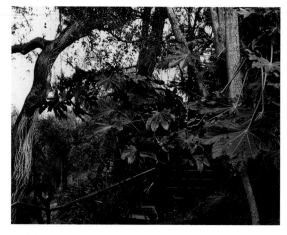

BOTANICAL NAME: *Feijoa sellowiana*
COMMON NAME: **PINEAPPLE GUAVA**
USDA ZONES: 8
ORIGIN: Paraguay, Southern Brazil, Argentina
FORM: Woody evergreen broadleaf shrub or tree
DESCRIPTION: Green glossy leaves, tomentose underneath, 2" to 3" long, oval in shape, pinnate veins
FLOWER COLOR: White, purple, 1-1/2" wide, red stamens, blooms from late spring to early summer
EXPOSURE: Full sun
WATER: Moderate
GROWTH RATE: Moderate
CHARACTERISTICS: Fruit is edible, tasting somewhat like kiwi, also high in vitamin C. Fruit takes 4 to 6 months to ripen sometimes longer in cooler climates. Expect fruit from September to December. Attracts bees and birds. Tolerates heat, drought conditions, reflected light and heat.
USES: Fruit, screen, hedge, espalier, multi-stemmed tree, and accent.

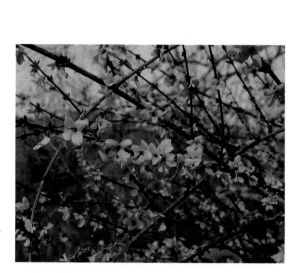

BOTANICAL NAME: *Forsythia intermedia*
COMMON NAME: **ARNOLD DWARF, FORSYTHIA**
USDA ZONES: 4, 5, 6, 7, 8, 9, 10
ORIGIN: East Asia
FORM: Woody deciduous arching broadleaf shrub, up to 10' tall
DESCRIPTION: Green leaves, up to 5" long, round in shape, pointed at the tip
FLOWER COLOR: Yellow, blooms from late winter to spring
EXPOSURE: Full sun
WATER: Moderate
GROWTH RATE: Fast
CHARACTERISTICS: Plant flowers on bare branches in late winter followed by a flush of leaves. This variety does not have spectacular flowers. Good in cold climates. Other varieties which produce attractive flowers are 'Beatrix Farrand,' 'Karl Sax.'
USES: Bank cover, screen, fast growing ground cover, accent, and cut flower.

BOTANICAL NAME: *Fuchsia hybrida*
COMMON NAME: **HYBRID FUCHSIA**
USDA ZONES: 6, 7, 8, 9, 10
ORIGIN: Parent plants from South America
FORM: Semi-herbaceous evergreen to deciduous arching broadleaf shrub, up to 20' long
DESCRIPTION: Light to dark green leaves, 3" long, opposite, ovate in shape, serrate margins
FLOWER COLOR: Red, pink, blue, white, variable size, blooms mostly in summer
EXPOSURE: Shade or heavy filtered sun
WATER: Regular and moist
GROWTH RATE: Fast
CHARACTERISTICS: Long and spectacular bloomer, prune back in late winter to revitalize, tip pinch to keep compact during flowering. Flowers have no fragrance, but do attract hummingbirds. Propagates readily from cuttings. Shade tolerant. Spray for mites and thrip. Leaf veins are reddish.
USES: Hanging baskets are most popular. Great for accenting a shady area. Other uses include accent, cut flower, espalier, ground cover, filler, and planter. Check varieties for specific uses.

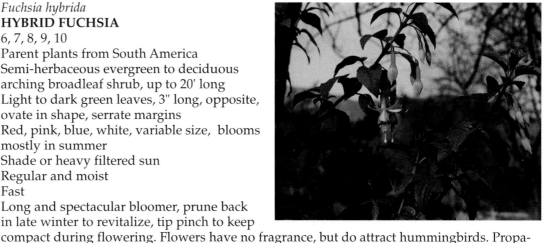

BOTANICAL NAME: *Gelsemium sempervirens*
COMMON NAME: **CAROLINA JESSAMINE**
USDA ZONES: 9
ORIGIN: Southeastern United States
FORM: Woody twining evergreen broadleaf vine, up to 20' long
DESCRIPTION: Light green glossy leaves, dull underneath, 1" to 4" long, attached to streamer-like branches
FLOWER COLOR: Yellow-gold, 1-1/2" long, tubular-shaped, blooms late winter to early spring
EXPOSURE: Full sun to partial shade
WATER: Moderate
GROWTH RATE: Moderate
CHARACTERISTICS: All parts are poisonous. Can get top heavy so prune back severely after flowering to lighten the load and untangle or lightly prune to keep in proper shape and size as desired. Fertilize after pruning. Moderately drought tolerant.
USES: Trellis, fences (including wrought iron fences), bank cover, and espalier.

BOTANICAL NAME: *Hakea suaveolens*
COMMON NAME: **SWEET HAKEA**
USDA ZONES: 9
ORIGIN: Australia
FORM: Woody evergreen broadleaf shrub, 10' to 20' tall
DESCRIPTION: Dark green leaves, simple, divided into needle-like lobes with spines, stiff, young foliage is holly-like
FLOWER COLOR: White, small, dense, fragrantly blooms from late fall to winter
EXPOSURE: Full sun
WATER: Infrequent, dry
GROWTH RATE: Medium to fast
CHARACTERISTICS: Leaves distinctive. Drought tolerant, grows well in coastal and hot arid conditions. Can be pruned into a tree form.
USES: Barrier, screen, hedge, and background. Very compatible with conifers.

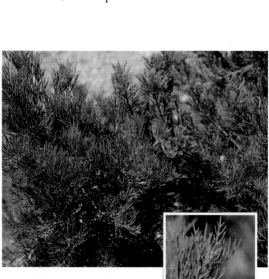

BOTANICAL NAME: *Hardenbergia comptoniana*
COMMON NAME: **VINE LILAC**
USDA ZONES: 9
ORIGIN: Australia
FORM: Woody evergreen broadleaf vine, up to 10' tall
DESCRIPTION: Dark green leaves, 2" to 3" long, narrow in shape, looks delicate, divided into 3 to 5 leaflets
FLOWER COLOR: Blue-violet, 1/2" wide, pea-shaped, in clusters, blooms from late winter to early spring
EXPOSURE: Full sun to partial shade
WATER: Low
GROWTH RATE: Moderate
CHARACTERISTICS: Needs well-drained soil, do not over water. Spray for spider mites. Plant beneath overhang where temperatures get below 24˚F to protect flower buds. Provide support when grown as a climbing vine. Provide partial shade in hot climates.
USES: Use in lacy areas as a climbing vine, archway, and on a fence. Can be used as a light screen.

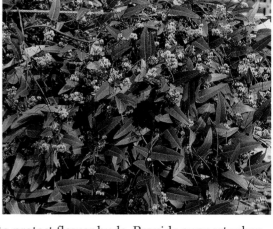

BOTANICAL NAME: *Heteromeles arbutifolia*
COMMON NAME: **CALIFORNIA HOLLY**
USDA ZONES: 7, 8, 9
ORIGIN: Sierra Nevada foothills and coast range in California, Baja California in Mexico
FORM: Woody evergreen dense broadleaf shrub, 6' to 10' tall, or tree 15' to 25' tall
DESCRIPTION: Green glossy leaves, leathery texture, 3" to 4" long by 1" to 2" wide, thick, prominent veins, serrate margins, red petioles
FLOWER COLOR: White, 3/16" long, in small clusters, blooms in mid-summer
EXPOSURE: Full sun to partial shade
WATER: Low to moderate
GROWTH RATE: Slow to moderate
CHARACTERISTICS: California native, drought tolerant. Flowers giveway to bright red berries from November to January. Prune to produce more berries or to train into small tree. Can be susceptible to fireblight.
USES: Winter color, cut foliage, decoration, native or Spanish setting, screen, and roadway.

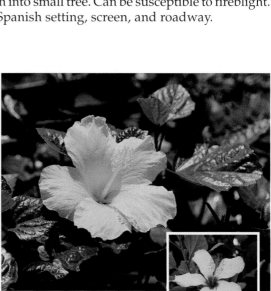

BOTANICAL NAME: *Hibiscus rosa-sinensis*
COMMON NAME: **CHINESE HIBISCUS**
USDA ZONES: 10, 11
ORIGIN: China
FORM: Woody evergreen broadleaf shrub or small tree, up to 15' tall
DESCRIPTION: Dark green glossy leaves, 4" to 6" long by 2" to 3" wide, simple, serrate margins
FLOWER COLOR: Red, white, pink, orange, yellow, apricot, 6" to 8" wide, tubular in shape, blooms in summer
EXPOSURE: Full sun
WATER: Regular and moist
GROWTH RATE: Moderate to fast
CHARACTERISTICS: Prune or thin yearly to promote perennial flowering, fertilize after pruning, keep soil acidic. Tolerates the heat, can't tolerate frost, coastal conditions or alkali soil. Provide good drainage.
USES: Oriental setting, summer color, accent, screen, terrace, and container.

BOTANICAL NAME: *Hydrangea macrophylla*
COMMON NAME: **GARDEN HYDRANGEA**
USDA ZONES: 5, 6, 7, 8, 9
ORIGIN: Japan
FORM: Woody deciduous broadleaf shrub, 4' to 8' tall
DESCRIPTION: Dark green leaves, 6" to 9" long by 3" to 6" wide, elliptic in shape, distinctive midrib, serrate margins
FLOWER COLOR: White, pink, red, blue, 6" to 10" wide, in large clusters, blooms from summer to fall
EXPOSURE: Full sun to partial shade in hot areas
WATER: High, keep moist
GROWTH RATE: Fast
CHARACTERISTICS: Prune in winter to remove old flower stems and rejuvenate. Flower color will change depending on the soil pH. Red or pink hydrangeas will turn blue when subjected to acidic soils. Blue or purple hydrangeas will turn red when subjected to neutral or basic soils.
USES: Accent, color, background, planter, container, and floral arrangement.

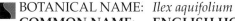

BOTANICAL NAME: *Ilex aquifolium*
COMMON NAME: **ENGLISH HOLLY**
USDA ZONES: 7, 8, 9
ORIGIN: British Isle, South-Central Europe
FORM: Woody evergreen broadleaf shrub or small tree, 20' to 40' tall
DESCRIPTION: Dark green leaves, usually 2" to 3" long, varies in shape, spines on margins
FLOWER COLOR: Inconspicuous, blooms from fall to winter, matures into red berries
EXPOSURE: Full sun to partial shade
WATER: Moderate to high
GROWTH RATE: Slow
CHARACTERISTICS: Protect from hot sun. Prefers acidic soils, however, will grow in basic soils if properly conditioned. Male and female plant are needed for the female to produce the red berries. Prune to shape and keep small. Resistant to oak root fungus. Variegated forms available.
USES: Small tree, large shrub, espalier, screen, formal or informal hedge, and winter berries.

BOTANICAL NAME: *Lantana camara*
COMMON NAME: **COMMON LANTANA**
USDA ZONES: 8, 9, 10
ORIGIN: North and South America
FORM: Woody evergreen to half deciduous trailing broadleaf shrub, 2' to 6' tall
DESCRIPTION: Dark green leaves, rough in texture, 2" to 3" long, ovate in shape, prominent veins
FLOWER COLOR: Red, orange, yellow, 1" to 2" wide, in clusters, blooms from spring to summer
EXPOSURE: Full sun, partial shade
WATER: Low to moderate
GROWTH RATE: Moderate to fast
CHARACTERISTICS: Prune yearly to rejuvenate and remove rattiness. Do not over fertilize or plant will not bloom very well. Tolerates many soil types and pH. Foliage is aromatic. Flowers all year in mild winter areas. Can survive on infrequent watering.
USES: Color, bank stabilizer, low informal hedge, ground cover, container, and rock garden.

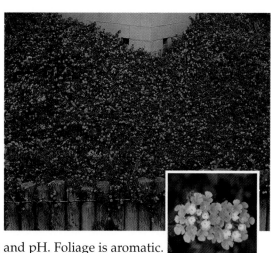

BOTANICAL NAME: *Laurus nobilis*
COMMON NAME: **SWEET BAY, GRECIAN LAUREL**
USDA ZONES: 8, 9, 10, 11
ORIGIN: Mediterranean area
FORM: Woody evergreen broadleaf shrub or tree, 10' to 40' tall
DESCRIPTION: Dark green leaves, leathery texture, 2" to 4" long, oval to oblong in shape
FLOWER COLOR: Yellow, 1/2" wide, in clusters, blooms in spring, matures into purple-black berries
EXPOSURE: Full sun to partial shade
WATER: Moderate at first, infrequent once established
GROWTH RATE: Slow
CHARACTERISTICS: Tolerates most soils if provided good drainage. Prune to control height and keep in bush form. Susceptible to black scale. Leaves aromatic when crushed.
USES: Screen, hedge, and background shrub. Leaves used in cooking.

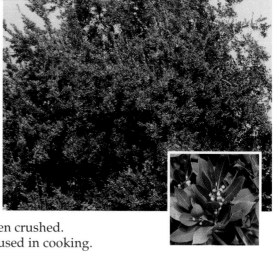

BOTANICAL NAME: *Leptospermum scoparium*
COMMON NAME: **NEW ZEALAND TEA TREE**
USDA ZONES: 9
ORIGIN: New Zealand, Australia
FORM: Woody evergreen mounding broadleaf shrub or ground cover, 1' to 10' tall
DESCRIPTION: Green dull leaves tinged with red, 1/2" long, simple, lanceolate in shape, looks lacy, aromatic
FLOWER COLOR: Red, white, pink, 1/2" wide, blooms in spring and summer
EXPOSURE: Full sun
WATER: Moderate, low once established
GROWTH RATE: Moderate
CHARACTERISTICS: Virtually pest free. Can become chlorotic in alkaline soils. Prune to shape and control size. Tolerates coastal conditions. Very showy in bloom.
USES: Hedge, tall ground cover, mass planting, screen, flower color, and filler.

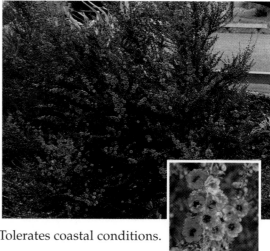

BOTANICAL NAME: *Mahonia aquifolium*
COMMON NAME: **OREGON GRAPE**
USDA ZONES: 5, 6, 7, 8, 9, 10
ORIGIN: Northern California to British Columbia
FORM: Woody evergreen upright broadleaf shrub, up to 6' tall
DESCRIPTION: Green glossy to dull leaves (depends on specific form), turning purple-red in winter, 4" to 10" long, compound with 5 to 9 spiny leaflets, young foliage is bronze
FLOWER COLOR: Yellow, 2" to 3" wide, in clusters, blooms from late winter to early spring, matures into fruit
EXPOSURE: Full sun to partial shade
WATER: Moderate
GROWTH RATE: Moderate
CHARACTERISTICS: State flower of Oregon. Spreads by underground stems (rhizomes). Prune to control height. Edible blue-black fruit.
USES: Barrier, medium screen, container, woodland setting, mass planting, and foliage variation. Fruit is used in jellies.

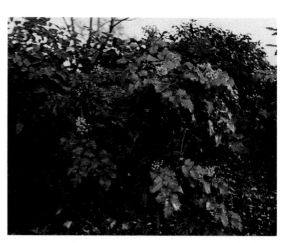

BOTANICAL NAME: *Mahonia pinnata*
COMMON NAME: **CALIFORNIA HOLLY GRAPE**
USDA ZONES: 8, 9,
ORIGIN: California, Southern Oregon
FORM: Woody evergreen upright broadleaf shrub, up to 8' tall
DESCRIPTION: Medium green leaves, wrinkly texture, 5" to 10" long, compound with 5 to 9 spiny leaflets, 1" to 1-1/2" long, oval in shape, young foliage is reddish-orange
FLOWER COLOR: Yellow, in clusters, blooms in spring
EXPOSURE: Full sun to partial shade
WATER: Moderate
GROWTH RATE: Moderate
CHARACTERISTICS: Will tolerate drought conditions once established. Prune to control height.
USES: Barrier, mass planting, woodland setting, foliage color, and colorful berries.

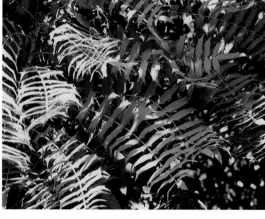

BOTANICAL NAME: *Myrtus communis 'Compacta'*
COMMON NAME: **DWARF MYRTLE**
USDA ZONES: 9
ORIGIN: Mediterranean area
FORM: Woody evergreen broadleaf shrub, up to 3' tall
DESCRIPTION: Green semi-glossy leaves, 1" long, ovate in shape, dense
FLOWER COLOR: White, 3/4" wide, fragrant, not very showy, blooms in summer
EXPOSURE: Full sun to partial shade
WATER: Moderate
GROWTH RATE: Slow
CHARACTERISTICS: Takes pruning very well. Can be shaped into a formal look. The leaves were once used as a symbol of peace and love. Leaves are aromatic when crushed.
USES: Small border, formal or informal hedge, topiary, filler, container, and bonsai.

BOTANICAL NAME: *Nandina domestica*
COMMON NAME: **HEAVENLY BAMBOO, NANDINA**
USDA ZONES: 6, 7, 8, 9
ORIGIN: India
FORM: Woody evergreen (semi-deciduous) broadleaf shrub, up to 8' tall
DESCRIPTION: Reddish-copper leaves in full sun, metallic blue leaves in shaded areas, 30" long, compound with numerous leaflets, 1/2" to 1" long, ovate in shape
FLOWER COLOR: White, in small clusters, not very showy, blooms from spring to early summer
EXPOSURE: Full sun to shade
WATER: Moderate
GROWTH RATE: Moderate
CHARACTERISTICS: Not actually considered part of the bamboo family. Colors are best if planted in full sun. Tolerant of drought conditions once established. Resistant to oak root fungus. Prune stalks to control height. Seedling grown plants are variable in growth habits where as tissue cultured plants are truer in growth habit.
USES: Oriental setting, container, tropical effect, near water, small area, and medium screen.

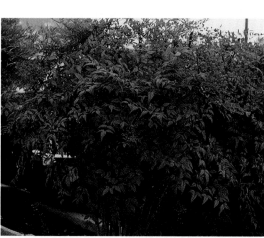

BOTANICAL NAME: *Passiflora edulis*
COMMON NAME: **PASSION FRUIT**
USDA ZONES: 7, 8, 9
ORIGIN: Brazil
FORM: Semi-evergreen sprawling broadleaf vine, 20' to 30' long
DESCRIPTION: Light green leaves, 2" to 3" long and wide, simple, margins deeply lobed in threes and serrate
FLOWER COLOR: White with purple crown, 2" to 3" wide, blooms in summer, matures into fruit
EXPOSURE: Full sun
WATER: Moderate
GROWTH RATE: Fast and vigorous
CHARACTERISTICS: Fruit is edible. Plant is very vigorous so cut back to main stem or branch on an annual basis after the second year in the ground. Will tolerate most types of soils. Fruitless varieties are available.
USES: Screen on a fence or wall. The fruit is used in fruit salads, beverages, and ice cream.

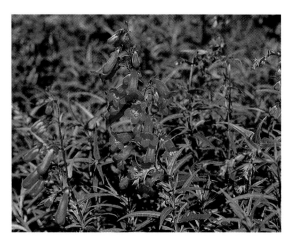

BOTANICAL NAME: *Penstemon gloxinioides*
COMMON NAME: **BORDER PENSTEMON**
USDA ZONES: 8, annual in colder climates
ORIGIN: California, Mexico
FORM: Herbaceous perennial broadleaf shrub, 2' to 4' tall
DESCRIPTION: Medium green leaves, 4" long, pointed at the tip, alternating up the stalks
FLOWER COLOR: Comes in many colors except yellow and blue, tubular spikes, blooms in summer
EXPOSURE: Full sun, partial shade in hot areas
WATER: Moderate to low
GROWTH RATE: Moderate
CHARACTERISTICS: Treated as an annual. Over watering can cause root rot in heavy soils. Cut back old blooms to flower again. Easily grown from seed or cuttings.
USES: Border, annual color, accent, mass planting, rock garden, and with other flowering summer annuals and perennials.

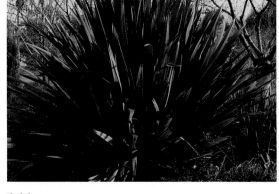

BOTANICAL NAME: *Phormium tenax*
COMMON NAME: **NEW ZEALAND FLAX**
USDA ZONES: 8
ORIGIN: New Zealand
FORM: Fibrous evergreen upright shrub, up to 9' tall
DESCRIPTION: Green leaves, up to 9' tall and 5" wide, spreading from base upward in a sword-like fashion
FLOWER COLOR: Reddish-yellow, 2" long, tall reddish stalks
EXPOSURE: Full sun to partial shade
WATER: Moderate
GROWTH RATE: Fast
CHARACTERISTICS: Allow plenty of room to grow. Very clean and vigorous plant. Will tolerate most any type of soil or exposure. Propagate by division. Bronze New Zealand Flax variety available.
USES: Wind break, background, near pool, foliage accent, medium focal point, and screen.

BOTANICAL NAME: *Photinia fraseri*
COMMON NAME: **PHOTINIA**
USDA ZONES: 8, 9, 10
ORIGIN: Hybrid cross
FORM: Woody evergreen broadleaf shrub or small tree, up to 15' tall
DESCRIPTION: Dark green glossy leaves, 2" to 4" long by 1-1/2" to 2-1/2" wide, elliptic in shape, alternating on the stem, serrate margins, young foliage is bronzy-red
FLOWER COLOR: White, 2" to 4" wide, in clusters, blooms from spring to early summer
EXPOSURE: Full sun
WATER: Moderate
GROWTH RATE: Moderate
CHARACTERISTICS: Prune out stems to control height and keep compact. Aphids can be a problem. Watch for chlorosis especially in alkaline soils. Will tolerate hot weather conditions and most any kind of soil. Shearing not recommended on this plant.
USES: Foliage accent, medium screen, informal hedge, espalier, planter, background, and large filler.

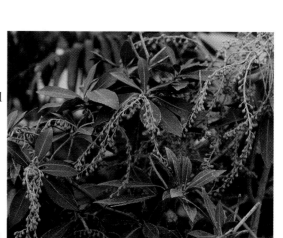

BOTANICAL NAME: *Pieris japonica*
COMMON NAME: **LILY-OF-THE-VALLEY SHRUB**
USDA ZONE: 5, 6, 7, 8
ORIGIN: East Asia, Himalayas, North America
FORM: Woody evergreen broadleaf shrub, 8' to 10' tall
DESCRIPTION: Dark green leaves, 3" long, young foliage is bronzy-red
FLOWER COLOR: White, pink, red, 1/4" to 3/8" long, attached to drooping stocks, blooms from late winter to early spring
EXPOSURE: Full shade to partial shade
WATER: High
GROWTH RATE: Moderate
CHARACTERISTICS: Protect from the wind. Provide good drainage so salts will not built up in soil. Responds well to fertilization.
USES: Specimen, flower color, and background shrub in woodsy or oriental setting. Good in large planter and entryway.

BOTANICAL NAME: *Pinus mugo mugo*
COMMON NAME: **MUGO PINE**
USDA ZONES: 3, 4, 5, 6, 7, 8
ORIGIN: Swiss Alps
FORM: Woody evergreen coniferous shrub, up to 4' tall and as wide
DESCRIPTION: Dark green needles, 1" to 2" long, stiff, closely set, in fascicles of 2
FLOWER COLOR: Inconspicuous, matures into pine cones
EXPOSURE: Full sun to partial shade
WATER: Moderate
GROWTH RATE: Very slow
CHARACTERISTICS: Dense compact shrub spreading with age. Very predictable slow grower. Not one to out grow or overtake an area. Very hardy for colder climates.
USES: Compact shrub, woodsy setting, low barrier, small planter, patio, rock garden, and understory.

BOTANICAL NAME: *Pittosporum eugenioides*
COMMON NAME: **TARATA**
USDA ZONES: 8
ORIGIN: New Zealand
FORM: Woody evergreen broadleaf shrub or tree, up to 40' tall
DESCRIPTION: Yellow-green semi-glossy leaves, 2" to 4" long by 1" wide, undulate margins
FLOWER COLOR: Yellow, 1/2" long, fragrant, blooms in spring
EXPOSURE: Full sun to partial shade
WATER: Moderate and regular
GROWTH RATE: Fast
CHARACTERISTICS: Prune out the top to keep in shrub form or selectively prune out undesired limbs to produce a medium large tree. Susceptible to aphids, scale, and sooty mold.
USES: Accent, foliage, shade tree, large planter, and large shrub.

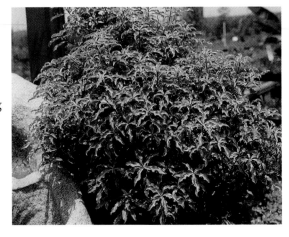

BOTANICAL NAME: *Pittosporum tobira*
COMMON NAME: **MOCK ORANGE**
USDA ZONES: 8
ORIGIN: China, Japan
FORM: Woody evergreen broadleaf shrub or small tree, 6' to 15' tall
DESCRIPTION: Green glossy leaves, leathery texture, 2-1/2" to 5" long by 1" wide, revolute margins
FLOWER COLOR: White, 1/2" wide, fragrant, blooms in early summer
EXPOSURE: Full sun to partial shade
WATER: Moderate
GROWTH RATE: Moderate
CHARACTERISTICS: Prune to keep small and compact, but do not over prune. Susceptible to scale and the usually accompanying sooty mold. Variegated form available and more commonly used in the landscape. Generally a clean plant. Variegated form has white leaf margins. Smells like orange blossoms.
USES: Good near pool, background, filler, planter, and foliar color.

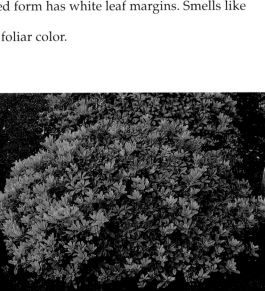

BOTANICAL NAME: *Pittosporum tobira 'Wheeler's dwarf'*
COMMON NAME: **WHEELER TOBIRA, MOCK ORANGE**
USDA ZONES: 8
ORIGIN: China, Japan
FORM: Woody evergreen broadleaf shrub, 1' to 2' tall
DESCRIPTION: Dark green leaves, leathery texture, 2" to 4" long by 1" wide, thick, round at the tip, revolute margins
FLOWER COLOR: Off-white, 1/2" wide, in small clusters, fragrant, blooms in early spring
EXPOSURE: Full sun to partial shade
WATER: Moderate until established, low thereafter
GROWTH RATE: Slow
CHARACTERISTICS: Drought resistant once established. Dependable, clean shrub. Used primarily for its foliage. Moderately susceptible to black scale and cottony cushion scale. Branches are brittle and break off easily so take care when planting and protect from animals.
USES: Small boundary shrub, ground filler, mass planting for tall ground cover effect, and near pool.

BOTANICAL NAME: *Plumbago capensis*
COMMON NAME: CAPE PLUMBAGO
USDA ZONES: 8
ORIGIN: South Africa
FORM: Evergreen to semi-evergreen sprawling broadleaf shrub, 8' to 12' tall and as wide
DESCRIPTION: Light green leaves, 1" to 2" long, pointed at the tip, in sets along arching branches
FLOWER COLOR: Powdery-blue, 1-1/2" wide, in clusters, blooms in summer
EXPOSURE: Full sun best
WATER: Moderate until established, low thereafter
GROWTH RATE: Moderate to fast
CHARACTERISTICS: Likes well draining soil. Does not bloom well if over watered or when planted away from full sun, so provide warm sunny location. Pinch back spent blooms to promote new blooms. Prune out selective stems in late winter to control size. Subject to nematodes. New growth subject to frost. Good in any hot location such as southern and western exposure.
USES: Half-hearted climber, filler, flower color, bank cover, and background plant.

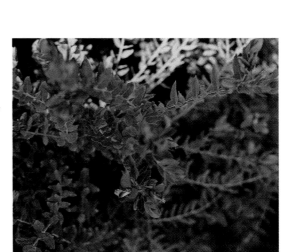

BOTANICAL NAME: *Polygala dalmaisiana*
COMMON NAME: SWEET-PEA SHRUB
USDA ZONES: 9
ORIGIN: Hybrid
FORM: Woody evergreen spreading broadleaf shrub, 2' to 5' tall
DESCRIPTION: Medium green leaves, 1" long, narrow in shape
FLOWER COLOR: Purple-pink, irregular shapes, attached to stalks, blooms almost continuously
EXPOSURE: Full sun to partial shade
WATER: Moderate
GROWTH RATE: Moderate
CHARACTERISTICS: Flowers sweet pea-like. Hard to color coordinate with other flowers. Prune to keep compact and control legginess. Long blooming period in spring and summer.
USES: Temporary color, filler, accent, and good in containers where plants can be moved when not in color.

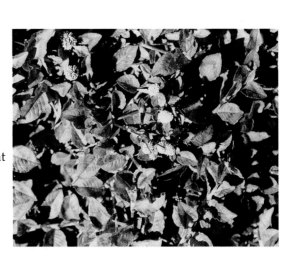

BOTANICAL NAME: *Polygonum capitatum*
COMMON NAME: ROSE CARPET KNOTWEED
USDA ZONES: 8
ORIGIN: Himalayas
FORM: Evergreen perennial prostrate broadleaf shrub or ground cover, 2' to 4' tall
DESCRIPTION: Green glossy leaves, turning red in fall, 1/2" long, oval in shape,
FLOWER COLOR: Rose-pink, 5/16" wide, densely set on upright stalks, blooms in late summer
EXPOSURE: Full sun
WATER: Moderate, higher in summer months
GROWTH RATE: Moderate
CHARACTERISTICS: Can get out of hand if not properly cared for, prune to control size. Needs frequent summer watering.
USES: Rock garden, amongst large boulders, bank cover, filler, color, and accent.

BOTANICAL NAME: *Punica granatum*
COMMON NAME: **POMEGRANATE**
USDA ZONES: 8, 9
ORIGIN: Southwest Asia
FORM: Woody deciduous broadleaf shrub or small tree, up to 12' tall
DESCRIPTION: Bright green glossy leaves, turning spectacular yellow in fall, 2" to 3" long, narrow in shape, young foliage is bronze
FLOWER COLOR: Red-pink, yellow, 2" to 4" wide, blooms in summer
EXPOSURE: Full sun
WATER: Moderate
GROWTH RATE: Moderate
CHARACTERISTICS: Grows well in alkaline soils. Tolerates a good deal of heat. Needs full sun for best flowers and fruit. Fruit is edible. Be careful of the thorns on the branches.
USES: Fruit is used in jellies. Flowers can be used in a corsage or as a cut flower. Good fall color plant.

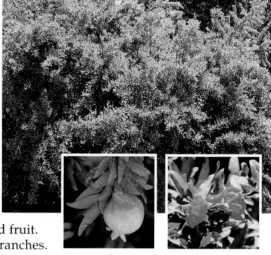

BOTANICAL NAME: *Rhaphiolepis indica*
COMMON NAME: **INDIAN HAWTHORN**
USDA ZONES: 8, 9
ORIGIN: Southern China
FORM: Woody evergreen compact broadleaf shrub, 4' to 5' tall
DESCRIPTION: Deep green glossy leaves, lighter green underneath, leathery texture, 2" long, ovate in shape, pointed at the tip
FLOWER COLOR: Whitish-pink, 1/2" wide, blooms from fall to late spring, matures into bluish-purple berries
EXPOSURE: Full sun best, partial shade okay
WATER: Moderate
GROWTH RATE: Moderate
CHARACTERISTICS: Flower color between varieties varies widely. Aphids can be a minor problem. Will adapt to a wide range of watering situations including drought. Avoid overhead irrigation if possible.
USES: Border, seasonal color (flowers and berries), filler, and planter.

BOTANICAL NAME: *Rhododendron spp.*
COMMON NAME: **RHODODENDRON**
USDA ZONES: 4, 5, 6, 7, 8, 9
ORIGIN: Northern Hemisphere, Himalayas, Asia
FORM: Woody evergreen and deciduous broadleaf shrubs, 2' to 25' tall
DESCRIPTION: Light to dark green leaves, 3" to 4" long by 1-1/2" to 2" wide (varies with variety)
FLOWER COLOR: Shades of white, pink, red, blue, various sizes, blooms from spring to early summer
EXPOSURE: Full sun in cooler summer areas, partial shade elsewhere
WATER: Moderate and frequent
GROWTH RATE: Moderate to semi-fast
CHARACTERISTICS: Over 10,000 varieties. Amend soils to achieve an acidic and porous condition. Plant rootball slightly higher than the soil level. Fertilize in spring and add phosphorus to improve blooming. Doesn't like clay and alkaline soils.
USES: Spectacular color in mass planting. There is a variety for almost any situation.

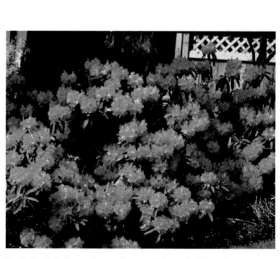

BOTANICAL NAME: *Ribes viburnifolium*
COMMON NAME: **CATALINA CURRANT**
USDA ZONES: 8, 9
ORIGIN: Baja California in Mexico, Catalina Island off the coast of California
FORM: Woody evergreen arching broadleaf shrub, up to 3' tall by 12' wide
DESCRIPTION: Dark green leaves, leathery texture, 1" long, round in shape, red stems, fragrant when crushed
FLOWER COLOR: Light pink to purple, small, blooms from late winter to spring, matures into fruit
EXPOSURE: Full sun to partial shade
WATER: Moderate until established, low thereafter
GROWTH RATE: Moderate
CHARACTERISTICS: Flowers and fruit attracts birds. Drought tolerant. Fragrant foliage.
USES: Good tall ground cover, bank cover, and stabilizer. A good choice near oak trees.

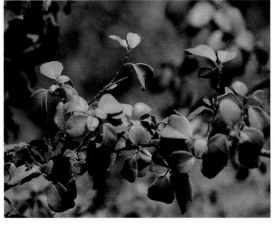

BOTANICAL NAME: *Romneya coulteri*
COMMON NAME: **MATILIJA POPPY**
USDA ZONES: 6, 7, 8, 9, 10
ORIGIN: Mexico, Southern California
FORM: Semi-woody evergreen broadleaf shrub, up to 8' tall
DESCRIPTION: Light blue silvery leaves, 3" to 4" long, satin-looking, cleft margins
FLOWER COLOR: White with yellow center, 4" to 9" wide, wrinkly, fragrant, blooms in late spring and summer
EXPOSURE: Full sun
WATER: Moderate until established, low thereafter
GROWTH RATE: Moderate, (depends on the amount of water given)
CHARACTERISTICS: Does not transplant well. Blooms on new wood, so prune after flowers have faded. Drought tolerant, but does better with moderate water. Will tolerate higher amounts of water as well.
USES: Somewhat course looking, best used in an out-of-the-way situation such as background shrub, bank, hillside, and roadside. Flowers used in floral arrangements.

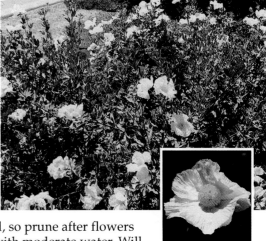

BOTANICAL NAME: *Sollya heterophylla (fusiformis)*
COMMON NAME: **AUSTRALIAN BLUEBELL CREEPER**
USDA ZONES: 9
ORIGIN: Australia
FORM: Spreading evergreen broadleaf shrub or vine, 2' to 3' tall
DESCRIPTION: Light green glossy leaves, 1" to 2" long, narrow in shape, attached to wiry stems
FLOWER COLOR: Blue, 1/2" long, bell-shaped, blooms in summer
EXPOSURE: Full sun, partial shade in hot areas
WATER: Moderate and regular
GROWTH RATE: Moderate
CHARACTERISTICS: Will reseed itself. Susceptible to nematodes and gophers. Provide good drainage.
USES: Good understory plant especially under eucalyptus trees. Good ground cover, container, and sprawling over low wall.

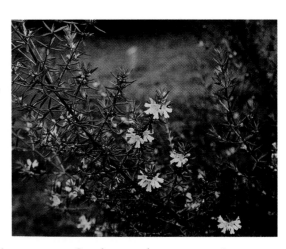

BOTANICAL NAME: *Spiraea bumalda 'Anthony Waterer'*
COMMON NAME: **DWARF RED SPIRAEA**
USDA ZONES: 5, 6, 7, 8, 9
ORIGIN: Hybrid
FORM: Woody deciduous dense shrub, up to 3' tall
DESCRIPTION: Green leaves tinged with dark red, 1" to 4" long, oval in shape
FLOWER COLOR: Red, small, in clusters, blooms from summer to fall
EXPOSURE: Full sun to partial shade
WATER: Moderate
GROWTH RATE: Moderate
CHARACTERISTICS: Many different varieties available. Adapts well in most soils. Prune in late winter. Snails and slugs can be a minor problem.
USES: Summer color, accent, border, foliage, cut flower, informal hedge, and old fashion garden.

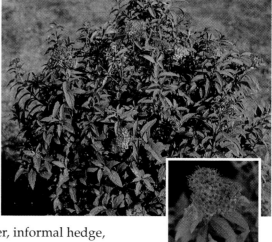

BOTANICAL NAME: *Strelitzia nicolai*
COMMON NAME: **GIANT BIRD OF PARADISE**
USDA ZONES: 9
ORIGIN: South Africa
FORM: Large tropical perennial shrub, up to 30' tall
DESCRIPTION: Gray-green leaves, leathery texture, 4' to 10' long (banana-like), thick, attached to erect curving trunks
FLOWER COLOR: Reddish-brown, white, dark blue, large, blooms all seasons, incidental
EXPOSURE: Full sun on coast, partial shade inland
WATER: Moderate and regular
GROWTH RATE: Moderate to fast
CHARACTERISTICS: Fertilize frequently (once a month) to reach mature size. Remove dead foliage and flowers. Thin out surplus growth. Not bothered by many pests.
USES: Great in tropical setting, near pool or pond, and indoor with tall ceiling and good light. Good in combination with banana tree (*Musa spp.*).

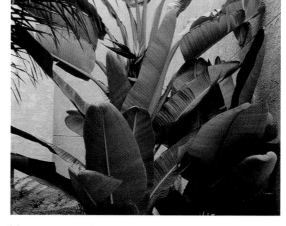

BOTANICAL NAME: *Strelitzia reginae*
COMMON NAME: **BIRD OF PARADISE**
USDA ZONES: 9
ORIGIN: South Africa
FORM: Tropical perennial shrub, 3' to 10' tall
DESCRIPTION: Green leaves, leathery texture, 1' to 2' long (banana-like but smaller), thick, curving upward on basal stalks
FLOWER COLOR: Orange, blue, white, 6" long, blooms mostly in spring, but can bloom anytime
EXPOSURE: Full sun on coast, partial shade elsewhere
WATER: Moderate and regular
GROWTH RATE: Moderate to fast
CHARACTERISTICS: Frost sensitive. Damage can occur when temperatures fall below 29˚ F. Flowers last about one month and can be forced to bloom. Blooms best in a crowded clump which takes 2 to 3 years after planting. Provide good drainage.
USES: Great in tropical setting, accent, specimen, flower color, container, planter, indoor near bright window, cut flower, and near pool, pond or other bodies of water.

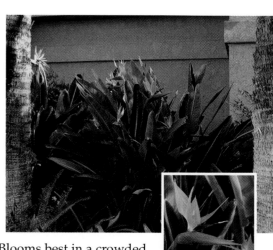

BOTANICAL NAME: *Symphoricarpos albus*
COMMON NAME: **COMMON SNOWBERRY**
USDA ZONES: 4
ORIGIN: North America
FORM: Woody deciduous upright or spreading broadleaf shrub, 2' to 6' tall
DESCRIPTION: Green dull leaves, 3/4" to 2" long, round in shape, sometimes lobed
FLOWER COLOR: Pink, 1/4" long, blooms from early summer to fall, matures into white fruit
EXPOSURE: Full sun to partial shade
WATER: Moderate until established
GROWTH RATE: Moderate
CHARACTERISTICS: Fruit attracts birds and remains on plant after leaves fall. Tolerant of poor soils, drought, poor air quality, shade and neglect. Fruit not as prominent in shady conditions.
USES: Thick tall ground cover, erosion control, poor air quality areas, understory, and woodsy setting.

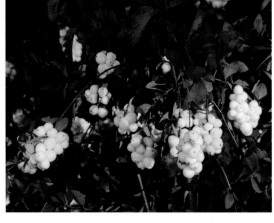

BOTANICAL NAME: *Syzygium paniculatum*
COMMON NAME: **AUSTRALIAN BRUSH-CHERRY**
USDA ZONES: 9, 10
ORIGIN: Australia
FORM: Woody evergreen large broadleaf shrub or small tree, 12' to 30' tall, 60' tall if untrimmed
DESCRIPTION: Dark green glossy leaves, lighter green underneath, 2" to 3" long by 1" wide, oblong to lanceolate in shape, young foilage is bronzy-red
FLOWER COLOR: Creamy-white, 1/2" long, blooms in summer, matures into rose-purple 3/4" fruit
EXPOSURE: Full sun to partial shade
WATER: Moderate to high
GROWTH RATE: Fast
CHARACTERISTICS: Fruit can be messy. Will not tolerate heavy frost. Needs good drainage. Can be trained into a single or multi-stemmed tree. Bronzy-red foliage makes for an attractive contrast.
USES: Large shrub, tree, hedge, columnar shrub, screen, and colored foliage.

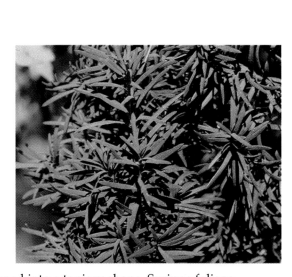

BOTANICAL NAME: *Taxus baccata*
COMMON NAME: **ENGLISH YEW**
USDA ZONES: 5, 6, 7, 8, 9
ORIGIN: Europe, Africa, Asia
FORM: Woody evergreen coniferous shrub or tree, 25' to 40' tall
DESCRIPTION: Dark green needles, light green underneath, 3/4" to 1-1/2" long, sickle in shape, flat, needle-like
FLOWER COLOR: Inconspicuous
EXPOSURE: Full sun to partial shade
WATER: Moderate and regular
GROWTH RATE: Slow
CHARACTERISTICS: Can tolerate high amounts of moisture and heavy pruning. Long lived plant. Seeds are poisonous. Transplants easily and can be pruned into a topiary shape. Syringe foliage occasionally in summer. Not bothered by pest or diseases. Somewhat drought tolerant.
USES: Hedge, screen, container, topiary, and specimen. Wood used in making long archery bows.

BOTANICAL NAME: *Tecomaria capensis*
COMMON NAME: **CAPE HONEYSUCKLE**
USDA ZONES: 9
ORIGIN: South Africa
FORM: Woody evergreen broadleaf shrub, 6' to 8' tall
DESCRIPTION: Dark green glossy leaves, 1/2" to 1" long by 3/4" wide, compound with 5 to 9 leaflets, rhomboid in shape, serrate margins
FLOWER COLOR: Orange-red to scarlet, 2" wide, tubular in shape, blooms from fall to winter
EXPOSURE: Full sun to partial shade
WATER: Low but regular
GROWTH RATE: Very fast
CHARACTERISTICS: Will tolerate some drought, wind, heat, and coastal conditions. Fertilize lightly once a year. Prune back far after flowering to maximize next year's blooms. Surface roots can be invasive. Susceptible to aphids and scale.
USES: Informal hedge, filler, espalier, barrier, semi-vine or ground cover, bank cover, and hot area.

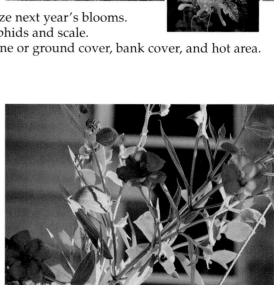

BOTANICAL NAME: *Tibouchina urvilleana (semidecandra)*
COMMON NAME: **PRINCESS FLOWER**
USDA ZONES: 9
ORIGIN: Brazil
FORM: Semi-woody evergreen irregular and spreading broadleaf shrub, 5' to 18' tall
DESCRIPTION: Dark green leaves, velvety texture, 3" to 6" long, oval in shape, ribbed veins, tinged with red margins, new growth and branch tips tainted with orange and bronzy-red hairs
FLOWER COLOR: Purple, 3" wide, in clusters, blooms from early summer to winter
EXPOSURE: Full sun, shade roots
WATER: Moderate
GROWTH RATE: Fast and open growth
CHARACTERISTICS: Protect from strong wind. Eastern or warmer exposures best. Needs acidic soil. Prune after blooms have faded to prevent legginess. Fertilize lightly after pruning. Remove tobacco bud worms if found; they can cause damage to the flower bud and prevent them from opening.
USES: Entryway, patio, container, indoor, border, tropical setting, and high humidity place.

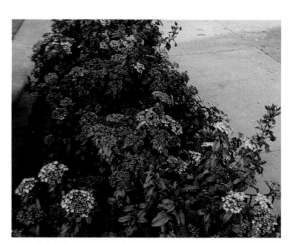

BOTANICAL NAME: *Viburnum spp.*
COMMON NAME: **VIBURNUMS**
USDA ZONES: 3, 4, 5, 6, 7, 8
ORIGIN: Mediterranean areas, Asia
FORM: Woody evergreen broadleaf shrub or small tree, 6' to 12' tall
DESCRIPTION: Dark green glossy leaves, pubescence underneath, leathery texture, 2" to 3" long by 1-1/2" wide, oval in shape, revolute margins, new stems are wine-red
FLOWER COLOR: White, pink buds, various sizes, usually in clusters, mildly fragrant, blooms in winter
EXPOSURE: Full sun
WATER: Moderate and regular
GROWTH RATE: Slow to moderate
CHARACTERISTICS: Fruit metallic blue throughout the summer. Susceptible to mildew near the coast.
USES: Screen, informal hedge, background, winter flower color, and small tree.

BOTANICAL NAME: *Weigela florida*
COMMON NAME: **WEIGELA**
USDA ZONES: 5, 6, 7, 8, 9
ORIGIN: Northern China, Korea
FORM: Woody deciduous mounding broadleaf shrub, up to 10' tall
DESCRIPTION: Medium to dark green leaves, slightly pubescence underneath, 2-1/2" to 3" long by 1-1/2" wide, semi-oval in shape, prominent veins
FLOWER COLOR: Pink to rose-red, 1-1/2" long, in clusters, blooms from late spring to summer
EXPOSURE: Full sun to partial shade
WATER: Moderate and regular
GROWTH RATE: Fast
CHARACTERISTICS: Tolerates air pollution, dust, smoke, reflected light, and cold. Spectacular display of spring color, but not very attractive plant out of bloom. Prune after flowering. Occasionally prune out old stems to the ground to stimulate new shoots.
USES: Screen, background, movable container, spring color, bank cover, and filler.

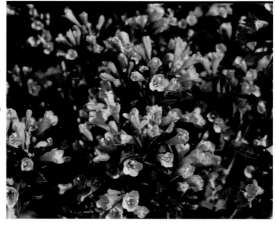

BOTANICAL NAME: *Xylosma congestum*
COMMON NAME: **SHINY XYLOSMA**
USDA ZONES: 8, 9
ORIGIN: Southeastern China
FORM: Woody evergreen broadleaf shrub or small tree, up to 25' tall
DESCRIPTION: Light to dark green glossy leaves tinged with bronzy-red, 3" to 5" long by 1" to 1-1/2" wide, oval in shape, pointed at the tip, slightly serrate margins
FLOWER COLOR: Inconspicuous
EXPOSURE: Full sun to partial shade
WATER: Moderate best, low summer water okay
GROWTH RATE: Moderate to fast
CHARACTERISTICS: Clean and attractive plant with its angular trunk and arching branches. Adapts to most soils. Drought tolerant once established but looks better with occasional water. Scale and spider mites can be a problem.
USES: Espalier, screen, small tree, filler, informal hedge, tall sprawling ground cover, and bank cover.

BOTANICAL NAME: *Yucca elata*
COMMON NAME: **SOAPTREE YUCCA**
USDA ZONES: 4, 5, 6, 7, 8, 9, 10
ORIGIN: Arizona, New Mexico, Texas
FORM: Fiberous evergreen shrub or small tree, 6' to 20' tall
DESCRIPTION: Green dull leaves, 4' long by 1/2" wide, sword-like in shape, tough, tips of leaves have a sharp spine
FLOWER COLOR: White, 2-1/2" long, on tall spikes, blooms in summer
EXPOSURE: Full sun
WATER: Moderate to infrequent
GROWTH RATE: Slow to moderate
CHARACTERISTICS: This is a desert plant so treat it like one. Drought tolerant once established. Well-drained soils best. Fire retardant. Spines can be dangerous so plant away from high traffic areas.
USES: Desert or cacti garden, near pool (not too close), and Spanish or chaparral setting.

BOTANICAL NAME: *Abies concolor*
COMMON NAME: **WHITE FIR**
USDA ZONES: 3, 4, 5, 6, 7
ORIGIN: Southern Oregon, California, Southwest United States, Baja California mountains in Mexico
FORM: Woody evergreen coniferous tree, up to 70' tall, and taller in its native environment
DESCRIPTION: Green dull needles, 1" to 2" long, in fascicles of 2, cones upright, 3" to 6" tall, barrel-shaped, young needles pale bluish-green
FLOWER COLOR: Inconspicuous, matures into cones
EXPOSURE: Full sun
WATER: Moderate
GROWTH RATE: Moderate to slow with age
CHARACTERISTICS: One of California's big lumber trees. Birds like to eat the seeds out of the cones. The leaves and buds are a source of winter food for some deer species. More readily available and most common of the fir trees, especially in the West. Conical in shape. Some dwarf forms are available. Insects and fungus can be a problem on older trees. Subject to limb and top breakage in high winds.
USES: Lumber, paper, Christmas tree, specimen, woodsy or alpine setting, accent, park, and cemetery.

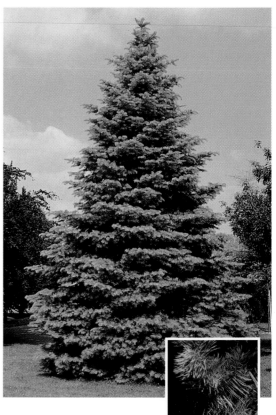

BOTANICAL NAME: *Abies grandis*
COMMON NAME: **GRAND FIR, LOWLAND FIR**
USDA ZONES: 5, 6, 7, 8
ORIGIN: British Columbia in Canada down the coast to Sonoma County in California, Idaho
FORM: Woody evergreen coniferous tree, up to 200' tall, much smaller out of its natural environment
DESCRIPTION: Green glossy needles, white stripes underneath, 1-1/2" to 2-1/4" long, in fascicles of 2
FLOWER COLOR: Inconspicuous, matures into cones
EXPOSURE: Full sun
WATER: Moderate
GROWTH RATE: Slow to moderate
CHARACTERISTICS: Very large fir tree and more attractive than most other firs. Birds like to eat the seeds. In the Northwest area people prune up the bottom limbs and successfully garden underneath them. Grand fir trees take on a conical shape.
USES: Specimen, accent, and native or alpine setting.

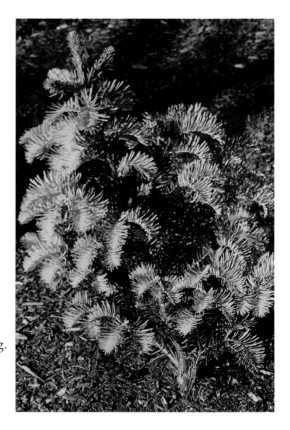

BOTANICAL NAME: *Albizia julibrissin*
COMMON NAME: **SILK TREE**
USDA ZONES: 6, 7, 8, 9, 10
ORIGIN: Iran, Japan
FORM: Woody deciduous broadleaf tree, mostly 10' to 20' tall, rarely 40' tall, umbrella-shaped
DESCRIPTION: Light green leaves, 10" to 12" long, compound with leaflets, 1/4" to 1/2" long, fern-like, sensitive to light, fold-up at night
FLOWER COLOR: Pink, 1-1/2 to 2" wide, puffy-looking, blooms in summer
EXPOSURE: Full sun
WATER: Moderate to high best, will survive on minimal watering
GROWTH RATE: Fast if properly watered
CHARACTERISTICS: Old-fashioned tree. Resembles the acacia tree. Distinctive form, light and airy. Does well in shallow or alkaline soils. Will also tolerate high water tables. Generally pest free, however, the spent flowers and seed pods can be messy. Stake when planted and prune to shape the first three years. The structure and form allows a lot of filtered sun light through the canopy.
USES: Light shade tree, lawn tree, summer color, patio tree (if you do not mind the seasonal mess), visual screen, and high altitude area.

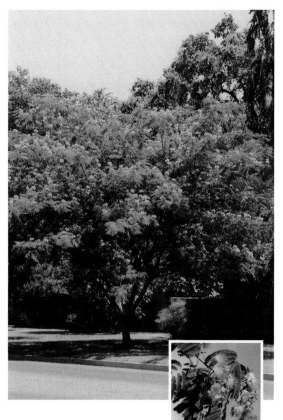

BOTANICAL NAME: *Arbutus unedo*
COMMON NAME: **STRAWBERRY TREE**
USDA ZONES: 7, 8, 9
ORIGIN: Southern Europe, Ireland
FORM: Woody evergreen irregular broadleaf small tree, 8' to 35' tall
DESCRIPTION: Dark green glossy leaves with red petioles, 2" to 4" long by 1" to 2" wide, serrate margins, dark brown twisting trunk
FLOWER COLOR: Cream-white to pinkish, 1/4" wide, bell-shaped, in clusters, blooms from fall to mid-winter, matures into red and yellow fruit
EXPOSURE: Full sun to partial shade
WATER: Moderate and regular best, drought tolerant once established
GROWTH RATE: Slow to moderate
CHARACTERISTICS: Tolerates some drought and adapts well to many different environments and soils, except alkaline soils. Red strawberry-like fruit, edible but rather bland tasting. Do not shear plant when pruning. Remove basal sprouts. Fertilize lightly in the spring with an acid forming fertilizer. Fruit drop can be messy so be careful where you plant it.
USES: Good near rocks, container, background plant, small tree, screen, and flower and fruit color. Can be used as a large shrub.

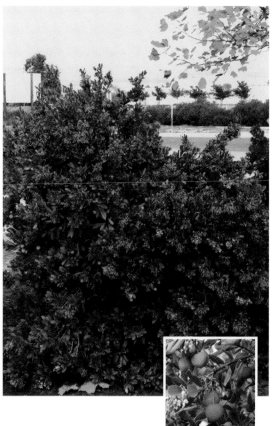

BOTANICAL NAME: *Bauhinia variegata*
COMMON NAME: **PURPLE ORCHID TREE**
USDA ZONES: 9
ORIGIN: China, India
FORM: Woody deciduous to semi-deciduous broadleaf tree or large shrub, 15' to 30' tall
DESCRIPTION: Gray green leaves, light pubescence underneath, leathery texture, 2" to 5" long, round in shape, lobed margins, notched on the tip, 7 to 11 nerved veins extending outward from the base of the leaf
FLOWER COLOR: Light pink to purple, 2" to 3" wide, fragrant, blooms from mid-winter to spring
EXPOSURE: Full sun
WATER: Moderate
GROWTH RATE: Moderate to fast
CHARACTERISTICS: Slightly resembles a redbud tree. Flowers appear the third year. Tolerates poor rocky soils and coastal conditions if protected from the wind. Somewhat messy flower drop. Will not tolerate cold temperatures. Scale, spider mites and mealybugs can be a problem as well as leaf spot fungus (in high humidity areas).
USES: Accent, flower color, specimen, lawn tree, and background. Looks good under night lighting.

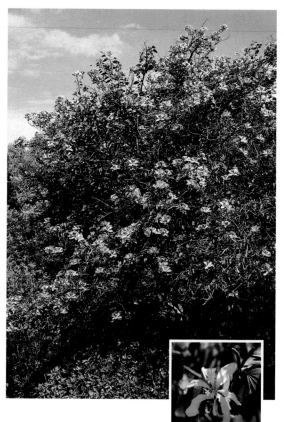

BOTANICAL NAME: *Brachychiton (Sterculia) populneus*
COMMON NAME: **BOTTLE TREE**
USDA ZONES: 9, best in 10, 11
ORIGIN: Queensland, New South Wales
FORM: Woody evergreen broadleaf tree, 30' to 50' tall by 30' wide
DESCRIPTION: Medium green glossy leaves, 2" to 3" long, pointed at the tip
FLOWER COLOR: White, small, in clusters, bell-shaped, not showy, blooms in late spring
EXPOSURE: Full sun
WATER: Low to moderate
GROWTH RATE: Moderate
CHARACTERISTICS: Trunks are unusually broad at the base tapering quickly. Looks similar to a poplar tree (*Populus*), but foliage more dense. Flowers are noticeable up close, but mostly used for its shimmering foliage. Can get Texas root rot if consistently over watered. Not recommended for lawn areas.
USES: Accent, moderate shade tree, desert setting, screen, windbreak, and areas of low or infrequent irrigation.

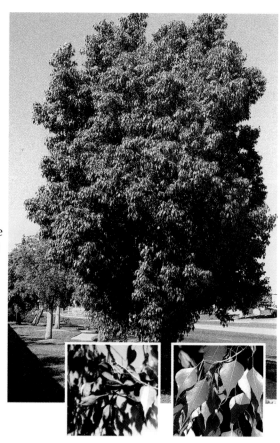

BOTANICAL NAME: *Catalpa speciosa*
COMMON NAME: **WESTERN CATALPA**
USDA ZONES: 5, 6, 7, 8, 9
ORIGIN: Southern Illinois south to Arkansas, Texas
FORM: Woody deciduous broadleaf tree, 40' to 60' tall
DESCRIPTION: Light green leaves, 8" to 12" long, heart-shaped
FLOWER COLOR: White with yellow and brown stripes, 2" wide, trumpet-shaped, blooms in late spring to summer.
EXPOSURE: Full sun
WATER: Moderate
GROWTH RATE: Moderate to fast
CHARACTERISTICS: Tolerates many extremes of heat, cold and soil types. Excellent flower color although somewhat hidden. Dead flowers and seed pods can be bothersome. Prune to shape while young to ensure a balanced tree.
USES: Shade tree, flower color, large specimen tree, background, and open space.

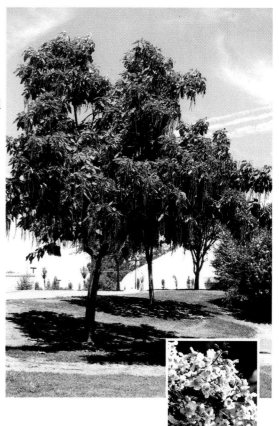

BOTANICAL NAME: *Celtis sinensis*
COMMON NAME: **CHINESE HACKBERRY**
USDA ZONES: 2, 3, 4, 5, 6, 7, 8, 9
ORIGIN: China, Korea, Japan
FORM: Woody deciduous broadleaf tree, 40' tall by 40' wide
DESCRIPTION: Bright green glossy leaves, 4" long, oval in shape, undulate margins, branches spreading and somewhat pendulous
FLOWER COLOR: Inconspicuous, matures into orange-red to dark purple fruit
EXPOSURE: Full sun
WATER: Moderate
GROWTH RATE: Moderate
CHARACTERISTICS: Related to the elm tree but smaller. Tolerates alkaline soils, heat, some wind and limited drought conditions. Young trees should be staked for 1 to 2 years. Resistant to oak root fungus. Late to leaf out in the spring. Deep rooted tree so uplifting is generally not a problem. (Bare root trees sometimes die before leaf break so make sure you get a guarantee from the seller).
USES: Narrow planter or small area, such as a parkway strip. Good near lawn or concrete walkway. Excellent wind-break or street tree.

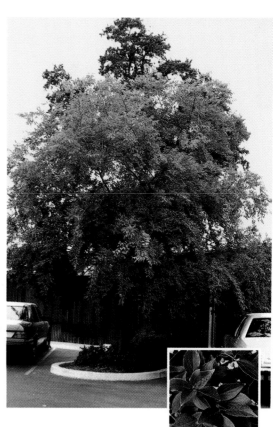

BOTANICAL NAME: *Cercis occidentalis*
COMMON NAME: **WESTERN REDBUD**
USDA ZONES: 4, 5, 6, 7, 8, 9
ORIGIN: California foothills, Arizona, Utah
FORM: Woody deciduous multi-trunk broadleaf small tree or large shrub, 12' to 18' tall
DESCRIPTION: Light green leaves turning yellow or red in fall, 3" to 5" long, round in shape, notched at the tip, leaves appear after flowers
FLOWER COLOR: Rosy to purplish-pink, 1/2" wide, pea-shaped, brilliant and bountiful clusters, blooms in spring, matures into seed pods in summer
EXPOSURE: Full sun to partial shade
WATER: Moderate until established (two years), then drought tolerant
GROWTH RATE: Moderate
CHARACTERISTICS: Great spring color. Drought resistant once established but does well with average garden watering. Resistant to oak root fungus. Prune out bottom stems to train into a small tree. Do not shear. Root system is deep, often tapping into underground water supplies. Flowers best when winter temperatures fall to at least 28° F.
USES: Bountiful spring color, native planting, infrequent watering area, and excellent understory shrub or tree.

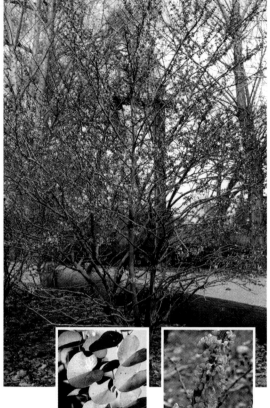

BOTANICAL NAME: *Chorisia speciosa*
COMMON NAME: **FLOSS-SILK TREE**
USDA ZONES: 9
ORIGIN: South America
FORM: Woody evergreen to slightly deciduous broadleaf tree, 30' to 60' tall
DESCRIPTION: Green leaves, palmately compound with 5 to 7 leaflets, lanceolate in shape, 4" to 6" long, serrate margins, trunk and branches have many sharp spines
FLOWER COLOR: Pink, white, purple-red to burgundy, 3" to 5" wide, showy, blooms from fall to early winter
EXPOSURE: Full sun
WATER: Moderate until established, about once a month thereafter
GROWTH RATE: Fast at first, then slow to moderate
CHARACTERISTICS: Do not water in late summer to maximize the tree's blooming potential. Be careful of the spines on the trunk. Remove if they pose a potential hazard. Tolerates heat, dry, humid or coastal conditions and some drought. Beautiful attractive flowers. Relatively pest free. Do not plant in lawn areas. White flowering species also available.
USES: Woodsy, prehistoric or Spanish setting. Good mixed with ferns, specimen, accent, and flowering tree.

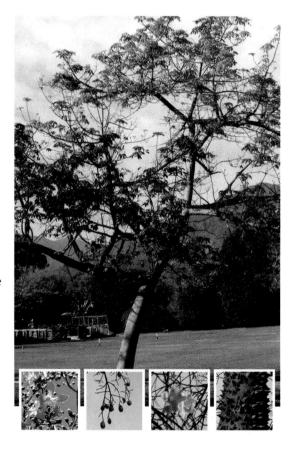

BOTANICAL NAME: *Cinnamomum camphora*
COMMON NAME: CAMPHOR TREE
USDA ZONES: 8, 9, 10
ORIGIN: Japan, China
FORM: Woody evergreen broadleaf tree, 40' to 50' tall and as wide
DESCRIPTION: Light green leaves, 2-1/2" to 5" long by 1" to 1-1/2" wide, oval to elliptic in shape, aromatic, young foliage tinged with bronzy-red
FLOWER COLOR: Inconspicuous, yellow, tiny, in clusters, fragrant, blooms in spring, matures into black fruit
EXPOSURE: Full sun
WATER: Moderate
GROWTH RATE: Moderate
CHARACTERISTICS: Likes hot summer climates. Crushed leaves smell like camphor. Root system can rise to the surface so do not plant in areas where uplifting would cause a problem, i.e. sidewalks, driveways, etc. Not bothered by any major pest, however, roots are susceptible to verticillium wilt if over watered or in areas of poor drainage. Expect a sizeable amount of leaf drop in the spring. All in all a good tree, just give it plenty of room to grow. Semi-messy.
USES: Shade tree, large specimen tree, and foliage color.

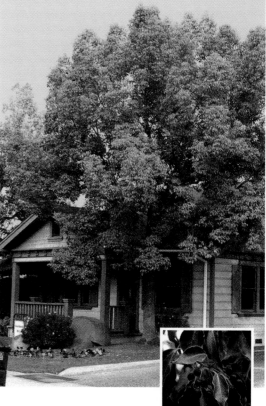

BOTANICAL NAME: *Cornus florida*
COMMON NAME: EASTERN DOGWOOD
USDA ZONES: 5, 6, 7, 9
ORIGIN: Eastern United States
FORM: Woody deciduous broadleaf small tree, up to 20' tall
DESCRIPTION: Light green leaves turning red in fall, 2-1/2" to 6" long by 2-1/2" wide, oval in shape
FLOWER COLOR: White, red, yellow, 2" to 4" wide, blooms in spring, matures into scarlet fruit
EXPOSURE: Shade to dappled shade, afternoon shade in hot areas
WATER: Moderate to high
GROWTH RATE: Slow to moderate
CHARACTERISTICS: Several cultivars available so check with your local nursery for the type you want. Branching habit is horizontal with upright tips. Profusion of flowers in the spring leading to small scarlet-colored fruit lasting well into the winter unless eaten by birds.
USES: Specimen tree, spring and fall color, patio tree, understory, movable container, and entryway.

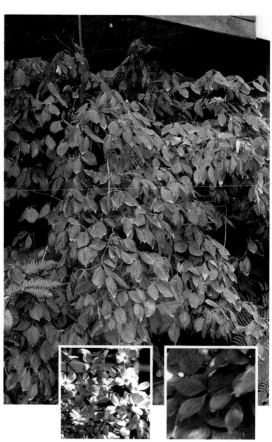

BOTANICAL NAME: *Cotinus coggygria*
COMMON NAME: SMOKE TREE
USDA ZONES: 5, 6, 7, 8
ORIGIN: Southern Europe
FORM: Woody deciduous broadleaf small tree, up to 25' tall
DESCRIPTION: Purple leaves turning yellow or red-orange in fall, 1-1/2" to 3" long, round to oval in shape
FLOWER COLOR: Yellow-green turning to a smokey-gray with purplish or greenish hairs 8" long, blooms from late spring to early summer
EXPOSURE: Full sun
WATER: Low to moderate, do not water in late summer
GROWTH RATE: Moderate
CHARACTERISTICS: Excellent fall colors. Flowers give off a purplish "smoke." Needs good draining soil if watered under "normal" garden conditions. Prune only when necessary, i.e., dead, diseased wood or crossing, hazardous limbs. Thrives in poor or rocky soils. Fruit is poisonous.
USES: Early summer color, native setting, drought or infrequent irrigated area (once established), fall color, and foliage accent.

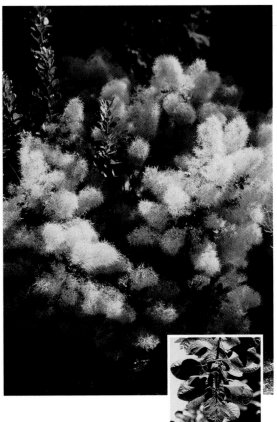

BOTANICAL NAME: *Cryptomeria japonica*
COMMON NAME: JAPANESE CRYPTOMERIA
USDA ZONES: 8, 9, 10
ORIGIN: Japan, China
FORM: Woody evergreen columnar coniferous tree, 40' to 60' tall
DESCRIPTION: Bright green leaves, 1/2" to 1"long, needle-like, young foliage tinged blue turning a brownish-purple in cold temperatures
FLOWER COLOR: Inconspicuous, matures into 1" wide cones
EXPOSURE: Full sun
WATER: Moderate to high
GROWTH RATE: Fast, 3' to 4' per year when young
CHARACTERISTICS: Several cultivars available, all smaller in size and slower growing (dwarf). Bark reddish-brown and peeling. Trunk straight and columnar. Cones reddish-brown. Resistant to oak root fungus. Needs deep soil.
USES: Skyline tree, background, oriental setting, and tall screen.

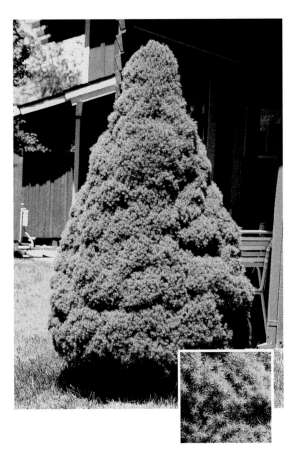

BOTANICAL NAME: *Eriobotrya deflexa*
COMMON NAME: BRONZE LOQUAT
USDA ZONES: 9
ORIGIN: Orient
FORM: Woody evergreen broadleaf small tree or large shrub, 10' to 20' tall
DESCRIPTION: Bronzy-red leaves turning green with age, leathery texture, 6" to 12" long by 3" wide, deeply veined, serrate margins, pointed at the tip
FLOWER COLOR: Creamy-white, 5/8" wide, blooms in spring, matures into fruit
EXPOSURE: Full sun partial shade
WATER: Moderate
GROWTH RATE: Fast
CHARACTERISTICS: Fruit not edible. Seems to be more resistant to fireblight than *Eriobotrya japonica*. Avoid reflected heat or southern exposures. Will take some drought once established.
USES: Small tree, specimen, container, foliage color, patio tree, and screen. Often used near brick work, wall, curb, and house.

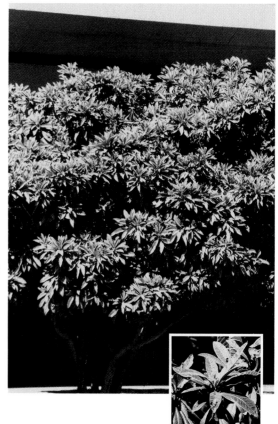

BOTANICAL NAME: *Eriobotrya japonica*
COMMON NAME: LOQUAT
USDA ZONES: 7, 8, 9
ORIGIN: Orient
FORM: Woody evergreen broadleaf small tree or large shrub, 15' to 25' tall
DESCRIPTION: Dark green glossy leaves, brown pubescence underneath, leathery texture, 6" to 12" long by 2" to 4" wide, deep veins, serrate margins
FLOWER COLOR: Inconspicuous, dull white, 3/8" to 3/4" wide, in clusters, blooms in fall, matures into fruit
EXPOSURE: Full sun to partial shade
WATER: Moderate
GROWTH RATE: Moderate to fast
CHARACTERISTICS: Fruit is edible and quite good. Thin out center to promote fruiting. Susceptible to fireblight. Thin out heavy bearing trees when fruit is young to allow remaining fruit to grow and ripen. Keep away from reflected heat. Flowers attract bees.
USES: Fruit tree, large shrub, screen, lawn tree, espalier on fence, container, and cut foliage for indoor arrangement.

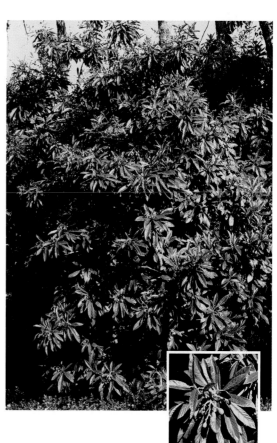

BOTANICAL NAME: *Erythrina bidwillii*
COMMON NAME: **CORAL TREE, BIDWILL CORAL**
USDA ZONES: 10
ORIGIN: Hybrid
FORM: Woody deciduous broadleaf small tree or large shrub, 8' to 20' tall and as wide
DESCRIPTION: Green leaves, compound into 3 broad ovate leaflets, middle leaflet is larger than the other two, many thorny branches
FLOWER COLOR: Red, 2" long, on 2' terminal stocks, blooms in summer
EXPOSURE: Full sun
WATER: Moderate and regular, keep moist in hot areas
GROWTH RATE: Fast
CHARACTERISTICS: Brilliant red mass of summer color. Tolerates coastal conditions and hot summer areas. Prune after flowers have faded. Very thorny so keep away from areas of high traffic such as sidewalks and entryways. Flowers can attract ants. Aphids can be a problem. Transplants well.
USES: Summer accent, flower color, screen, mass planting, specimen, background, and semi-tropical setting.

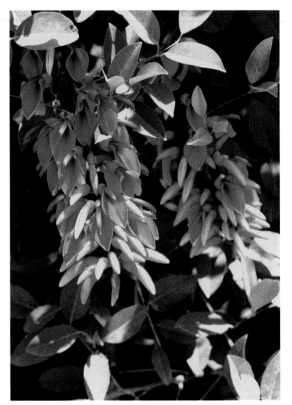

BOTANICAL NAME: *Eucalyptus cinerea*
COMMON NAME: **ARGYLE APPLE**
USDA ZONES: 9
ORIGIN: Australia
FORM: Woody evergreen broadleaf tree, 20' to 50' tall and as wide
DESCRIPTION: Mature ash-color leaves, 3" to 4" long, lanceolate in shape, juvenile gray-green leaves, 1" to 2" long, in pairs, round in shape
FLOWER COLOR: Inconspicuous, 3/8" long, blooms from early to late winter
EXPOSURE: Full sun
WATER: Moderate
GROWTH RATE: Fast
CHARACTERISTICS: Can become scrawny unless properly pruned. Growth habit is snake-like (twisting and curving). Plant in dryer areas or where drainage is good. Tolerates wind.
USES: Used mostly for juvenile foliage in flower arrangement, and sometimes as a specimen tree.

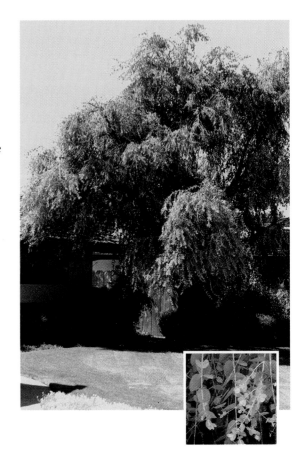

BOTANICAL NAME: *Eucalyptus sideroxylon*
COMMON NAME: **RED IRONBARK**
USDA ZONES: 9
ORIGIN: Australia
FORM: Woody evergreen broadleaf tree, 20' to 80' tall
DESCRIPTION: Green leaves tinged with blue turning bronze in winter, 4" to 6" long by 1/2" to 1" wide, narrow in shape
FLOWER COLOR: Creamy-white to rose, 3/4" long, in small clusters, blooms from fall to spring
EXPOSURE: Full sun
WATER: Moderate
GROWTH RATE: Moderate to fast
CHARACTERISTICS: Trunk very dark almost black. Bark furrowed and non-shedding making it one of the cleaner eucalyptus species. Growth characteristics vary widely between trees because they are grown from seed. Tolerates alkaline soils, wind, heat,drought, and coastal conditions.
USES: Screen, street tree, highway tree, winter flower color, background, specimen, and shade tree.

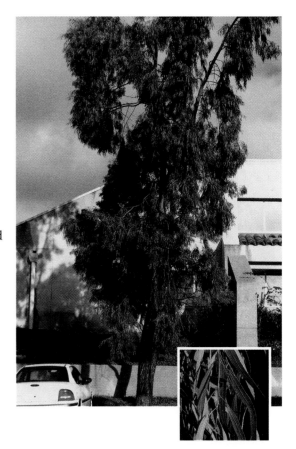

BOTANICAL NAME: *Ficus benjamina*
COMMON NAME: **WEEPING FIG, BANYAN TREE**
USDA ZONES: 9
ORIGIN: India, northern tropical Australia
FORM: Woody evergreen broadleaf small tree or large shrub, 15' to 30' tall and as wide
DESCRIPTION: Deep green glossy leaves, leathery texture, 2" to 5" long by 1" wide, elliptical in shape, pointed at the tip, undulate margins
FLOWER COLOR: Inconspicuous
EXPOSURE: Full sun to shade
WATER: Moderate and regular
GROWTH RATE: Moderate
CHARACTERISTICS: Does not like sudden changes in its environment (light intensity, temperature and humidity) especially when used as an indoor plant. Tolerates coastal conditions, low light and humidity. Will not tolerate wind, cold (frost) or close proximity to indoor air conditioner vents.
USES: Mostly used as a house plant or in indoor shopping malls. Other uses include container, shade tree, topiary, patio, and entryway.

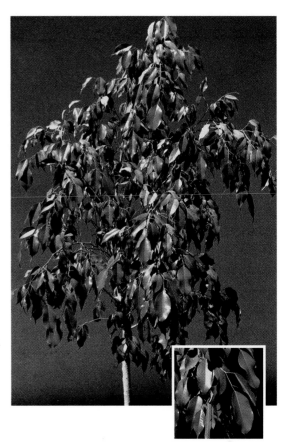

BOTANICAL NAME: *Fraxinus oxycarpa 'Raywood'*
COMMON NAME: **RAYWOOD ASH**
USDA ZONES: 6
ORIGIN: Hybrid
FORM: Woody deciduous rounded tree, up to 35' tall
DESCRIPTION: Deep green leaves, turning into deep purple-red to brown in fall, 5" to 10" long, compound with several leaflets with one terminal leaflet, narrow to lancelote in shape
FLOWER COLOR: Sterile, no flowers
EXPOSURE: Full sun
WATER: Moderate to high
GROWTH RATE: Fast
CHARACTERISTICS: This ash is a hybrid and does not produce flowers or pollen. It's the only ash considered allergy-free. Variable but great fall color of deep purple-red to brown. Roots are invasive so plant away from house, sidewalk, and sewer systems.
USES: Shade tree, fall color, quick growth, and perimeter planting.

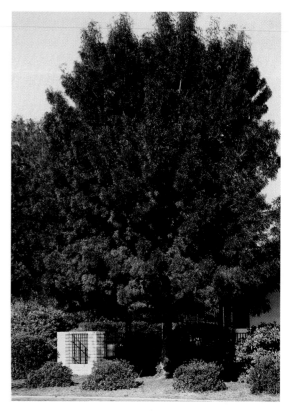

BOTANICAL NAME: *Ginkgo biloba*
COMMON NAME: **MAIDENHAIR TREE**
USDA ZONES: 3, 4, 5, 6, 7, 8, 9
ORIGIN: China
FORM: Woody deciduous broadleaf tree, 35' to 80' tall
DESCRIPTION: Green leaves turning yellow in fall, 2" to 4" wide, fan-shaped, notch at the tip, undulate margins, parallel veins
FLOWER COLOR: Inconspicuous
EXPOSURE: Full sun
WATER: Moderate and regular
GROWTH RATE: Slow when young, then moderate
CHARACTERISTICS: Truly a specimen tree. Virtually pest free. Particularly noted for its beautiful fall color. Leaves keep their color after they fall off the tree. It is common practice to leave the fallen leaves on the ground throughout the holidays. The only drawback is its slow growth and awkwardness when young. Ginkgo's are dioecious. Plant only in the male species. The female ginkgo tree produces a messy smelly fruit.
USES: Excellent fall color, specimen, lawn tree, mass planting, shade tree, and patio.

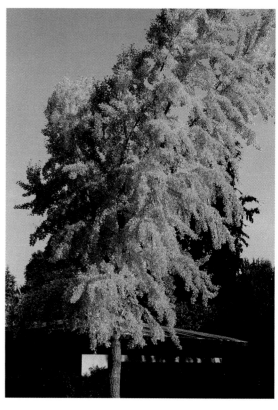

BOTANICAL NAME: *Gleditsia triacanthos inermis*
COMMON NAME: **HONEY LOCUST**
USDA ZONES: 3, 4, 5, 6, 7, 8, 9
ORIGIN: Eastern United States
FORM: Woody deciduous broadleaf tree, 35' to 70' tall
DESCRIPTION: Light green leaves, 10" long, compound with many leaflets, 3/4" to 1-1/2" long, oval in shape
FLOWER COLOR: Inconspicuous
EXPOSURE: Full sun
WATER: Moderate and regular
GROWTH RATE: Fast
CHARACTERISTICS: Open and airy tree. Good in lawns or where filtered shade is desired. Don't plant near foundations, sidewalks, curbs or septic systems. The root system is very aggressive and tends to be surface oriented. Susceptible to many pests including borers, pod midge gall, and mimosa webworm. Tolerant of many soils. Does best in climates with distinguishing winters and summers. Leafs out later in spring and drops off early in autumn.
USES: Lawn tree, light shade tree, mild accent, good middle ground tree with green shrubs below and taller green trees behind.

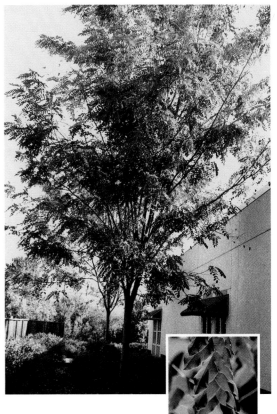

BOTANICAL NAME: *Grevillea robusta*
COMMON NAME: **SILK OAK**
USDA ZONES: 9
ORIGIN: Australia
FORM: Woody evergreen conical broadleaf tree, 30' to 60' tall
DESCRIPTION: Dark to golden green leaves, silvery underneath, 6" to 12" long, compound with numerous leaflets, fern-like
FLOWER COLOR: Orange (no petals), 2-3/4" long, in large clusters, blooms in early spring
EXPOSURE: Full sun
WATER: Low to moderate
GROWTH RATE: Fast
CHARACTERISTICS: Limbs are very brittle and break easily. The root system is very invasive so do not plant near sidewalks, driveways, or house foundations. Fast growing tree often used as a temporary quick shade tree until other more desirable trees mature then it is removed. Will tolerate poor compacted soils if not over watered. Also tolerant of drought, frost (to 16˚ F on established trees), and hot areas. High leaf drop in the spring. Somewhat messy tree. Aphids and scale can be a minor problem.
USES: Background tree, desert planting, quick growth, screen, and shade tree.

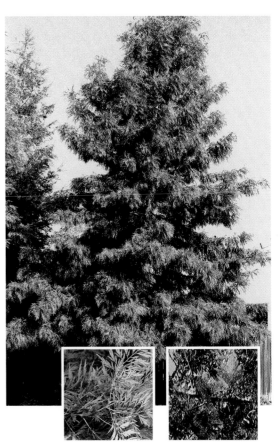

BOTANICAL NAME: *Jacaranda acutifolia*
COMMON NAME: **JACARANDA**
USDA ZONES: 9
ORIGIN: Brazil, Argentina
FORM: Woody semi-deciduous broadleaf tree, 25' to 45' tall
DESCRIPTION: Green leaves, 16" to 20" long, compound with 6 to 13 leaflets
FLOWER COLOR: Lavender, 2" long, tubular-shaped, in 8" long clusters, blooms from spring to fall, mostly in summer
EXPOSURE: Full sun to shade
WATER: Moderate
GROWTH RATE: Fast
CHARACTERISTICS: Tolerates heat, shady areas, and drought. Susceptible to aphids, scale and oak root fungus. Will not tolerate constantly wet soils, frost or wind. Can be somewhat messy.
USES: Accent, street tree, shade tree, patio tree, and flower color.

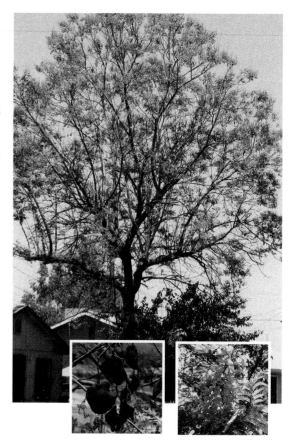

BOTANICAL NAME: *Koelreuteria paniculata*
COMMON NAME: **GOLDENRAIN TREE**
SUNSET ZONE: 5, 6, 7, 8, 9
ORIGIN: Japan, China, Korea
FORM: Woody deciduous broadleaf tree, 20' to 35' tall and as wide
DESCRIPTION: Green leaves in summer turning yellow in fall, 15" long, compound with 7 to 15 leaflets, 1" to 3" long, lobed in shape, young leaves purple-red
FLOWER COLOR: Yellow, 8" to 14" wide, in long clusters, showy, fragrant, blooms in summer, matures into fruit
EXPOSURE: Full sun
WATER: Moderate
GROWTH RATE: Slow to moderate
CHARACTERISTICS: Tolerates heat, wind, some drought, coastal conditions, alkaline soils, smoke, dust, and smog. Susceptible to oak root fungus. Not bothered by many pest. Attracts bees. Attractive brownish papery fruit shaped like an inverted rain drop 1-1/2" long, persist on the tree into the fall or winter.
USES: Street tree, patio tree, shade tree, accent, oriental or Spanish setting, and flowering tree.

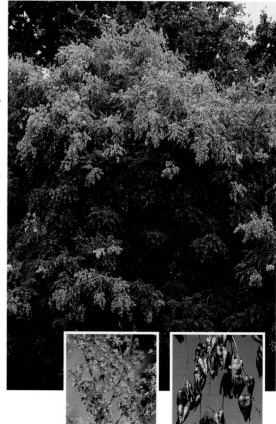

■ BOTANICAL NAME: *Lagerstroemia indica*
COMMON NAME: CRAPE MYRTLE
USDA ZONES: 7, 8, 9
ORIGIN: China, Korea, India
FORM: Woody deciduous broadleaf small tree or large shrub, 6' to 30' tall
DESCRIPTION: Green glossy leaves in spring turning bronzy-red in fall, 1" to 2-3/4" long by 1" wide, oblong to elliptic in shape
FLOWER COLOR: Pink, red, lavender, white, 1-1/2" wide, in crepe-like clusters, blooms in summer
EXPOSURE: Full sun
WATER: Low to moderate
GROWTH RATE: Slow
CHARACTERISTICS: Prune back in winter to promote flowering next spring and summer. Aphids are a problem and should be controlled to maximize the flowering potential. Can become chlorotic in alkaline soils. Loves hot climates and will take some drought.
USES: Small flowering tree, shrub, patio tree, container, street tree, hedge, and summer screen. Good against southern or western exposure wall.

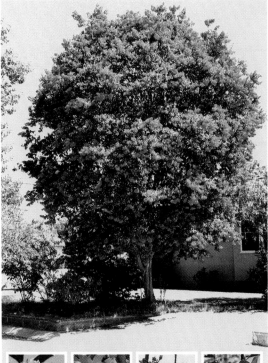

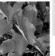

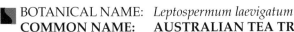

■ BOTANICAL NAME: *Leptospermum laevigatum*
COMMON NAME: AUSTRALIAN TEA TREE
USDA ZONES: 9
ORIGIN: Australia, New Zealand
FORM: Woody evergreen broadleaf small tree or large shrub, up to 30' tall
DESCRIPTION: Gray green leaves, 1" long by 3/8" to 1/2" wide, teardrop in shape
FLOWER COLOR: White, 1/2" wide, attached along the branches, blooms in spring
EXPOSURE: Full sun
WATER: Moderate until established, infrequent thereafter
GROWTH RATE: Moderate
CHARACTERISTICS: Does best in well-drained slightly acidic soils. Grows fine with little care. A very uniform looking tree with fine textured, weeping branches. As a tree, becomes very picturesque with a gray-brown, twisted trunk of irregular shape. Shrub forms need pruning to stay compact. Shrub forms also lose some of their gracefulness.
USES: Specimen tree, flowering tree, and shrub. Shrub form used as a wind break or shear into a flowering hedge.

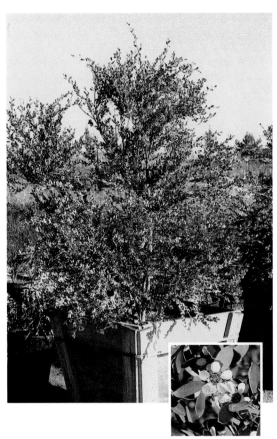

■ BOTANICAL NAME: *Liriodendron tulipifera*
COMMON NAME: TULIP TREE
USDA ZONES: 4, 5, 6, 7, 8, 9
ORIGIN: Eastern United States, Massachusetts, Wisconsin, Florida, Mississippi
FORM: Woody deciduous broadleaf tree, 60' to 80' tall by 40' wide
DESCRIPTION: Light green leaves turning yellow in the fall, 5" to 6" wide, end of the leaf truncate, two lobes at the base
FLOWER COLOR: Yellow-green and orange at the base, 2" wide (not easily seen), blooms in late spring
EXPOSURE: Full sun
WATER: Moderate and regular
GROWTH RATE: Fast
CHARACTERISTICS: Large tall tree so give it some room to grow. Good fall color and a great replacement for sycamore trees, especially in hot inland areas. Can get scale, aphids, and thrip. Flowers quite attractive but hard to see. No major disease problems.
USES: Shade tree, lawn tree, and fall color. Timber used for making furniture, and boats.

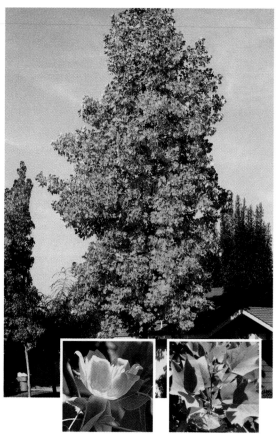

■ BOTANICAL NAME: *Magnolia grandiflora*
COMMON NAME: SOUTHERN MAGNOLIA
USDA ZONES: 6, 7, 8, 9
ORIGIN: North Carolina, Florida
FORM: Woody evergreen broadleaf tree, up to 80' tall and 40' wide
DESCRIPTION: Dark green glosssy leaves, sometimes rusty-red pubescence underneath, 4" to 8" long, oblong in shape, thick
FLOWER COLOR: White, 8" wide, attached to cone-like stalks, fragrant, blooms in summer and fall
EXPOSURE: Full sun to partial shade
WATER: Moderate until established, once a month thereafter
GROWTH RATE: Slow to moderate
CHARACTERISTICS: Tolerates heat and some wind. Large grand or majestic looking tree. Flowers are fragrant. Red seed drop just before new blooms appear. Can be messy all year long.
USES: Street tree, lawn tree, flower color, and southern or stately setting.

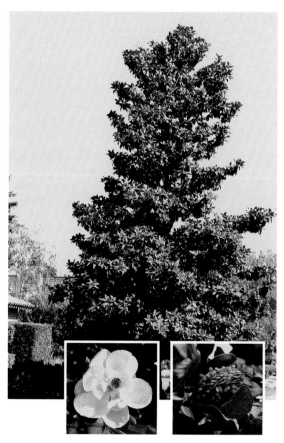

BOTANICAL NAME: *Magnolia soulangiana*
COMMON NAME: **SAUCER MAGNOLIA**
USDA ZONES: 5, 6, 7, 8, 9
ORIGIN: Hybrid
FORM: Woody deciduous broadleaf multi-stemmed tree, up to 25' tall
DESCRIPTION: Green dull leaves turning yellow and brown in fall, 5" long, narrow in shape
FLOWER COLOR: White to pink, 3" wide, numerous, fragrant, blooms in late winter and early spring
EXPOSURE: Full sun to shade
WATER: Moderate
GROWTH RATE: Slow
CHARACTERISTICS: Flowers before leaves appear. One of the first plants to bloom out of winter. Don't let the soil dry out. Protect from windy areas. Prefers acidic soils.
USES: Accent, specimen, excellent flower display for late winter, patio, container, and oriental or woodsy setting.

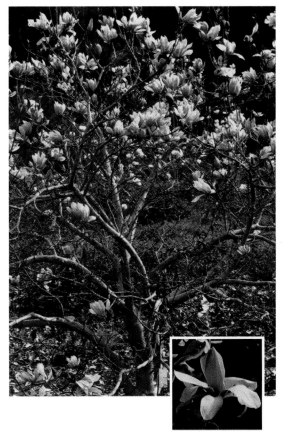

BOTANICAL NAME: *Maytenus boaria*
COMMON NAME: **MAYTEN TREE**
USDA ZONES: 8, 9
ORIGIN: Chile, Argentina
FORM: Woody evergreen broadleaf tree, 30' to 50' tall
DESCRIPTION: Medium green leaves, 1" to 2" long by 1/2" wide, narrow in shape, attached to long pendulous branches, fine serrate margins
FLOWER COLOR: Inconspicuous
EXPOSURE: Full sun to partial shade
WATER: Moderate and deep
GROWTH RATE: Slow to moderate
CHARACTERISTICS: Must have good drainage. Water deeply or roots will be shallow and promote suckers. Prune out undesirable side growth on the trunk. Can take some drought once established. Resembles a small scale weeping willow, but with more character. Resistant to oak root fungus.
USES: Excellent lawn tree (if watered deeply), street tree, specimen, entryway, patio tree, and small shade tree, near pool and ponds.

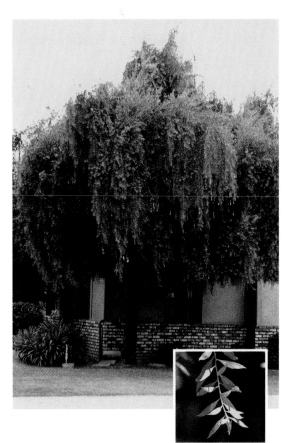

■ BOTANICAL NAME: *Archontophoenix cunninghamiana*
  COMMON NAME: **KING PALM, SOLITAIRE PALM**
  USDA ZONES: 9
  ORIGIN: Queensland, Australia, New South Wales
  FORM: Evergreen monoecious palm tree,
    50' to 80' tall by 15' wide
  DESCRIPTION: Medium green fronds, grayish underneath,
    8' to 10' long by 3' wide, feather-like,
    somewhat stiff looking blades
  FLOWER COLOR: Purple-red, 2" to 4" long, in hanging clusters,
    mildly fragrant
  EXPOSURE: Full sun to shade
  WATER: Moderate
  GROWTH RATE: Fast
  CHARACTERISTICS: Very clean and neat palm tree with virtually
    no disease or pests. Protect from strong winds.
    Established or large container trees do not
    transplant very well. Plant 15 gallon or smaller
    size for best results. Tolerates heat, coastal
    conditions and some drought. Old fronds
    shed cleanly from the trunk. Remove flower
    spikes early.
  USES: Tropical effect, street tree, patio palm, accent,
    container, and near pool (keep away from
    chlorinated pool water).

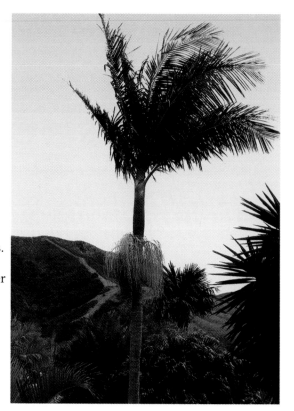

■ BOTANICAL NAME: *Arecastrum romanzoffianum*
  COMMON NAME: **QUEEN PALM, COCOS PALM**
  USDA ZONES: 9
  ORIGIN: Argentina to Brazil
  FORM: Evergreen monoecious palm tree, 30' to 50'
    tall by 25' to 30' wide
  DESCRIPTION: Medium green glossy fronds, 10' to 15' long
    by 4' to 6' wide, feather-like, arching graceful
  FLOWER COLOR: Inconspicuous, yellow-white, 2' to 3' long,
    in hanging clusters
  EXPOSURE: Full sun
  WATER: Moderate
  GROWTH RATE: Fast
  CHARACTERISTICS: Protect from strong winds. Tolerates
    coastal conditions, heat, humidity and some
    drought. Grows best with consistent water
    and semi-annual fertilizing. Susceptible to
    spider mites. Hose off foliage frequently.
    Remove flower spikes early and queen palms
    will be totally allergy-free. Fairly clean palm
    tree, and transplants easily.
  USES: Tropical effect, patio palm, street tree, accent,
    lining driveway, near pool and pond.

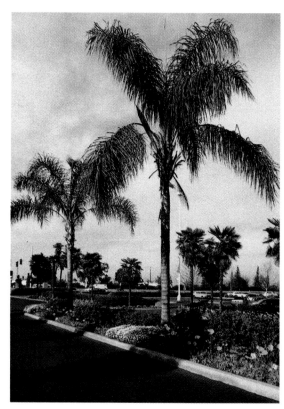

BOTANICAL NAME: *Brahea armata*
COMMON NAME: **MEXICAN BLUE PALM**
USDA ZONES: 9
ORIGIN: Baja California in Mexico
FORM: Evergreen monoecious palm tree, 25' to 40' tall by 6' to 10' wide
DESCRIPTION: Gray-blue to silvery-white fronds, 2' to 3-1/2' long by 6' wide, fan-like, curved sharp teeth on petiole
FLOWER COLOR: Creamy-white, 3' long, in large pendulous clusters
EXPOSURE: Full sun
WATER: Low, very drought tolerant
GROWTH RATE: Very slow
CHARACTERISTICS: One of the most drought tolerant of all palm trees available. Over watering can cause leaf tip burn especially in alkaline soils and root rot. Tolerates heat, wind, and arid conditions. Likes higher pH soils (pH 7.3 to 8.5) and good drainage. Noted mostly for its unusual leaf color. Growth rate may vary even when planted in groups in the same location.
USES: Tropical effect, specimen, accent, container, and areas of no added irrigation.

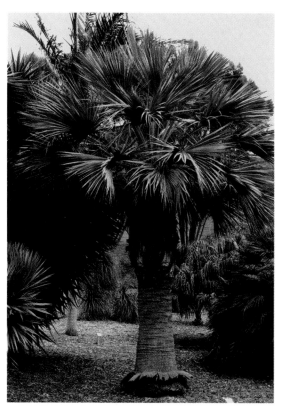

BOTANICAL NAME: *Chamaedorea elegans*
COMMON NAME: **PARLOR PALM**
USDA ZONES: 10, 11
ORIGIN: Mexico, Guatemala
FORM: Evergreen monoecious palm small tree, up to 4' tall
DESCRIPTION: Medium to dark green fronds, 3' to 5' long, feather-like, single stemmed palm
FLOWER COLOR: Inconspicuous
EXPOSURE: Partial shade to shade
WATER: Moderate and regular
GROWTH RATE: Very slow
CHARACTERISTICS: Excellent indoor palm. Needs good drainage and occasional fertilizing. Syringe foliage to keep clean and attractive. Remove dead or old dying leaves. Plant three in a container to produce a fuller interesting look. Repot every two years by replenishing the soil. Once a month slowly flush container with water for ten minutes to leach out harmful salt buildup.
USES: Mostly used indoors in homes, shopping malls and professional offices. Good entryway and patio palm.

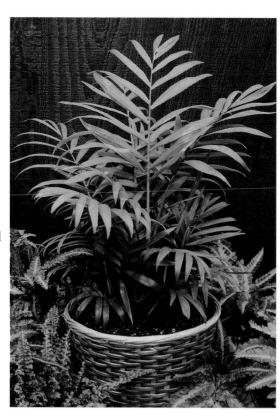

BOTANICAL NAME: *Chamaerops humilis*
COMMON NAME: MEDITERRANEAN FAN PALM
USDA ZONES: 9
ORIGIN: Greater Mediterranean area
FORM: Evergreen monoecious palm tree, 15' to 20' tall and eventually as wide
DESCRIPTION: Medium green fronds tinged with blue, 2' to 3' wide, stiff, fan-shaped, sharp spikes on the petiole
FLOWER COLOR: Yellow, in short clusters, blooms in spring
EXPOSURE: Full sun to partial shade
WATER: Moderate
GROWTH RATE: Slow to moderate
CHARACTERISTICS: Tolerates heat, drought, wind, arid conditions, acid or alkaline soils, and cold temperatures to 6° F. Fertilize in the summer months to increase growth rate. Avoid consistent soggy soil in the root zone or root rot might set in. Suckers can occur from base often producing a clustered interesting look. Remove undesirable suckers.
USES: Container, indoor and patio palm, tropical effect, and in a cluster.

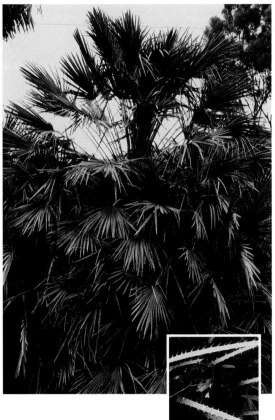

BOTANICAL NAME: *Phoenix roebelenii*
COMMON NAME: PIGMY DATE PALM
USDA ZONES: 9
ORIGIN: Loas, Vietnam, Southeast Asia
FORM: Evergreen small palm tree, 6' to 10' tall and as wide
DESCRIPTION: Dark green glossy fronds, fine texture, 4' long, feather-like, looks graceful, 3" thin spines on petiole
FLOWER COLOR: Inconspicuous
EXPOSURE: Partial shade to shade
WATER: Moderate and regular
GROWTH RATE: Slow
CHARACTERISTICS: Fine and delicate textured single trunk palm. Tolerates low light, some heat, and wind. Protect from the cold. Cross pollinates easily so buy from a reliable source. Relatively pest and disease free.
USES: Excellent for houses, malls, and offices (make sure that the spines are removed for safety, especially if young children are present). Other uses include patio palm, planter, entryway, accent, specimen, tropical setting, and near pool (remove spines).

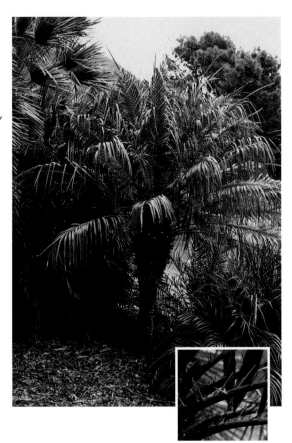

BOTANICAL NAME: *Trachycarpus fortunei*
COMMON NAME: **WINDMILL PALM, CHUSAN PALM**
USDA ZONES: 8
ORIGIN: Central and Eastern China, Burma
FORM: Evergreen palm tree, 20' to 30' tall by 10' to 20' wide
DESCRIPTION: Green dull fonds, 2' to 4' wide, fan-shaped, looks glaucous, long saw-toothed petioles
FLOWER COLOR: Inconspicuous
EXPOSURE: Full sun
WATER: Moderate
GROWTH RATE: Moderate
CHARACTERISTICS: Tolerates heat, some drought, wind, and cold temperatures to 10^0 F. Needs some care to look its best. Remove dead fronds and fertilize in summer. Trunk wrapped with fibrous sheaths and is wider at the top tapering down to the base. Fairly clean palm tree.
USES: Tropical effect, specimen, accent, patio palm, street tree, and container. Good above night lighting.

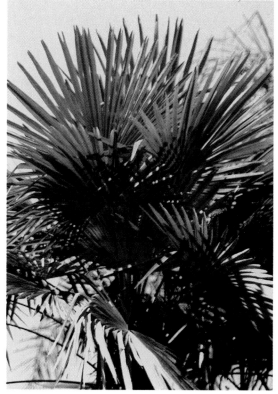

BOTANICAL NAME: *Washingtonia filifera*
COMMON NAME: **CALIFORNIA FAN PALM**
USDA ZONES: 9
ORIGIN: Arizona, Southern California
FORM: Evergreen palm tree, 60' tall by 25' wide
DESCRIPTION: Gray-green fronds, 3' to 6' wide, fan-shaped, long fibrous threads hang from fronds, sharp teeth on petiole, dead fronds remain on palm
FLOWER COLOR: White, blooms in spring
EXPOSURE: Full sun
WATER: Moderate and regular
GROWTH RATE: Moderate to fast
CHARACTERISTICS: Thick trunk to 3' in diameter. Tolerates heat, wind, and humidity. Remove dead fronds to keep neat, clean and to eliminate nesting place for mice and rats. Prevent soil from becoming consistently soggy in root area.
USES: Street, boulevard or avenue tree, tropical effect, accent, specimen, open space, and multiple planting. Attractive near water (if drainage is good).

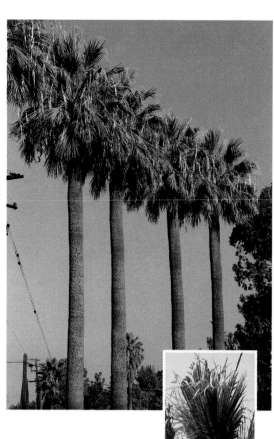

BOTANICAL NAME: *Washintonia robusta*
COMMON NAME: **MEXICAN FAN PALM**
USDA ZONES: 9
ORIGIN: Baja California in Mexico, Southern California
FORM: Evergreen palm tree, up to 100' tall
DESCRIPTION: Medium to dark green fronds, 4' to 8' long by 5' wide, fan-shaped, a few fibrous threads hang from fronds, short curved teeth on petiole
FLOWER COLOR: Inconspicuous
EXPOSURE: Full sun
WATER: Moderate and regular
GROWTH RATE: Fast to very fast
CHARACTERISTICS: Trunk very slender and slightly curving as it matures. Tolerates heat, wind, and some drought. It will do better with regular watering and care. Remove dead fronds to keep neat, clean, and to eliminate nesting place for mice and rats. More graceful looking than *Washingtonia filifera*.
USES: Skyline tree, street, avenue or boulevard tree, accent, specimen, background, tropical setting, group planting, and desert setting. Good near water (if drainage is good).

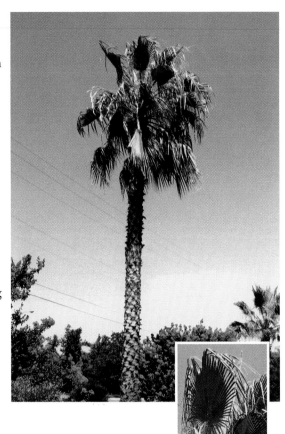

BOTANICAL NAME: *Pinus canariensis*
COMMON NAME: **CANARY ISLAND PINE**
USDA ZONES: 8, 9
ORIGIN: Canary Island near Spain
FORM: Woody evergreen coniferous tree, 60' to 80' tall by 40' wide
DESCRIPTION: Bright bluish-green to darker grayish-green needles, 9" to 12" long, in fascicles of 3, pendulous, needles live for about two years then fall-off
FLOWER COLOR: Inconspicuous, matures into pine cones
EXPOSURE: Full sun
WATER: Moderate, regular and deep
GROWTH RATE: Fast
CHARACTERISTICS: Stake when young for support. Tolerates heat and some drought, but does best with moderate watering, poor well-draining soils, and coastal conditions. Can get scale, twig borer, aphids, western gall rust. Resistant to oak root fungus. Slender and graceful in its youth, spreading out at maturity. Young trees seem a little gawky, but grow out of it relatively fast.
USES: Accent, avenue or mass planting, background, and woodsy setting.

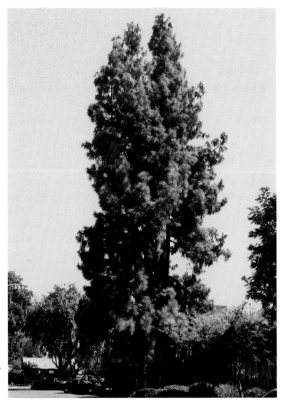

BOTANICAL NAME: *Pinus halepensis*
COMMON NAME: **ALEPPO PINE, JERUSALEM PINE**
USDA ZONES: 7
ORIGIN: France, Spain, Greece, Italy
FORM: Woody evergreen coniferous tree, 40' to 60' tall by 20' to 30' wide
DESCRIPTION: Yellow to light green needles, 2-1/4" to 4" long, in fascicles of 2, sometimes 3
FLOWER COLOR: Inconspicuous, matures into pine cones
EXPOSURE: Full sun
WATER: Low to moderate
GROWTH RATE: Slow at first then fast thereafter
CHARACTERISTICS: Tolerates heat, drought, neglect, alkaline soils, coastal conditions, and wind. Can get scale, bark beetles, needle minor, and stem blister rust. Can form a round headed tree.
USES: Windbreak, specimen, quick growth, shade tree, background, golf course, park, and desert condition.

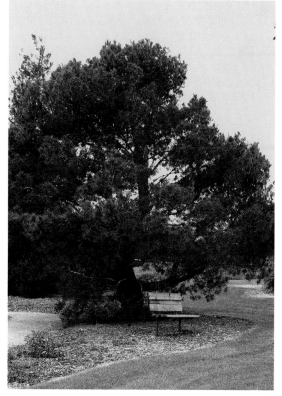

BOTANICAL NAME: *Pinus radiata*
COMMON NAME: **MONTEREY PINE**
USDA ZONES: 8
ORIGIN: California Central Coast
FORM: Woody evergreen coniferous tree, 80' to 100' tall
DESCRIPTION: Green needles, 4" to 7" long, in fascicles of 3, sometimes 2
FLOWER COLOR: Inconspicuous, matures into pine cones
EXPOSURE: Full sun
WATER: Moderate
GROWTH RATE: Fast to very fast
CHARACTERISTICS: Not tolerant of extreme hot or cold temperatures or smog. Lower branches fade as tree matures. Susceptible to spotted spider mite. Trees lean in areas of constant wind, and may fall over under strong windy conditions.
USES: Native coastal setting, wind break when young, mountainous setting, and shade.

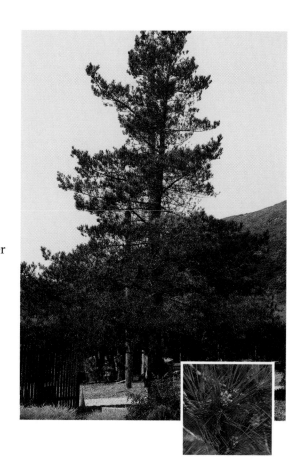

■ BOTANICAL NAME: *Pinus thunbergiana*
COMMON NAME: **JAPANESE BLACK PINE**
USDA ZONES: 5
ORIGIN: Japan
FORM: Woody evergreen coniferous tree, 20' to 100' tall (varies by region)
DESCRIPTION: Medium green needles, 4" to 5" long, stiff, sharply pointed, in fascicles of 2
FLOWER COLOR: Inconspicuous, matures into pine cones
EXPOSURE: Full sun
WATER: Moderate
GROWTH RATE: Fast in northern latitudes, slow in southern latitudes and deserts
CHARACTERISTICS: Tolerates city and coastal conditions, heat, and wind. Not tolerant of constantly wet or alkaline soils. Slow grower in lowland desert areas. Can get aphids, scale and twig borers. Open and airy tree.
USES: Accent, oriental setting, bonsai, patio, container, and planter.

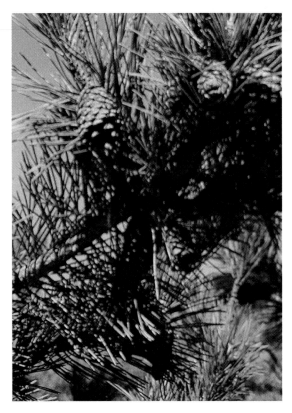

■ BOTANICAL NAME: *Pistacia chinensis*
COMMON NAME: **CHINESE PISTACHE**
USDA ZONES: 7, 8, 9
ORIGIN: China, Taiwan, Philippines
FORM: Woody deciduous broadleaf tree, 40' to 60' tall
DESCRIPTION: Medium green leaves in summer turning orange-yellow to scarlet in fall, compound with pairs of 6 to 10 leaflets, 2" to 4" long by 1/2" to 3/4" wide,
FLOWER COLOR: Inconspicuous
EXPOSURE: Full sun
WATER: Moderate
GROWTH RATE: Slow to moderate
CHARACTERISTICS: Excellent fall color. Will tolerate alkaline soils, some drought, and heat. Can get scale occasionally. Resistant to oak root fungus, but can become infected with verticillium wilt in soggy soils. Prune to shape when young, and stake if needed.
USES: Shade tree, fall color, street tree, lawn tree, patio, accent, and specimen.

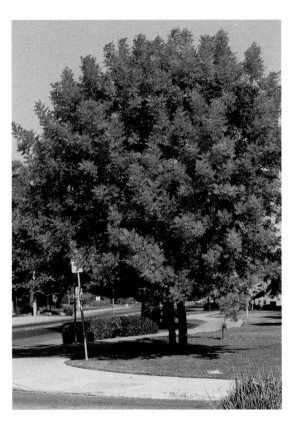

BOTANICAL NAME: *Podocarpus gracilior*
COMMON NAME: **FERN PINE, PODOCARPUS**
USDA ZONES: 9, 10
ORIGIN: East Africa
FORM: Woody evergreen coniferous tree or large shrub, up to 40' tall
DESCRIPTION: Bluish-green leaves, 1" to 2" long, narrow in shape, closely spaced, distinct midrib
FLOWER COLOR: Inconspicuous
EXPOSURE: Full sun to partial shade
WATER: Moderate
GROWTH RATE: Slow to moderate
CHARACTERISTICS: Takes pruning well. Prune into a columnar shrub or let grow into a tree. Not bothered by many pests except occasional aphids. Generally a very clean tree or shrub. Will grow indoors near outside light. Soft appearance.
USES: Patio, container, understory, topiary, hedge, and oriental setting.

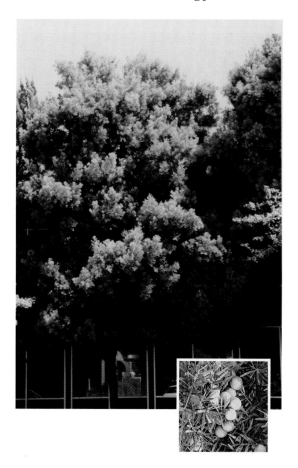

BOTANICAL NAME: *Podocarpus macrophyllus*
COMMON NAME: **YEW PINE, PODOCARPUS**
USDA ZONES: 8
ORIGIN: Japan
FORM: Woody evergreen coniferous tree or large shrub, up to 50' tall
DESCRIPTION: Deep green leaves, pale green underneath, 4" long by 1/2" wide, narrow in shape
FLOWER COLOR: Inconspicuous
EXPOSURE: Full sun to partial shade
WATER: Moderate
GROWTH RATE: Slow to moderate
CHARACTERISTICS: Does not like reflected light or heat. Leaves bigger than *Podocarpus gracilior* and more coarse looking. Will grow indoors near outside light. Mostly seen growing in a columnar fashion, but will grow free form.
USES: Patio, container, understory, entryway, hedge, screen, shady area, and near redwoods, maples or where a softer look is desired.

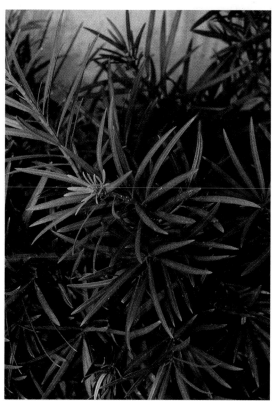

BOTANICAL NAME: *Prunus caroliniana*
COMMON NAME: **CAROLINA CHERRY**
USDA ZONES: 8
ORIGIN: North Carolina southwest to Texas
FORM: Woody evergreen broadleaf tree, up to 40' tall
DESCRIPTION: Green glossy leaves, 2" to 4" long by 1" to 2" wide, oblong in shape, young foliage bronzy-red
FLOWER COLOR: Creamy-white, 3/16" wide, attached to spikes, blooms from winter to early spring, matures into fruit
EXPOSURE: Full sun
WATER: Moderate
GROWTH RATE: Fast
CHARACTERISTICS: Do not plant near walks or where fruit drop will be a problem. Drought tolerant once established. Not tolerant of alkaline soils. Tolerates wind, heat, humidity, and coastal conditions. Prune to shape. Susceptible to brown scale and fireblight.
USES: Tall screen, background, windbreak, park, coastal planting, and hedge if pruned properly.

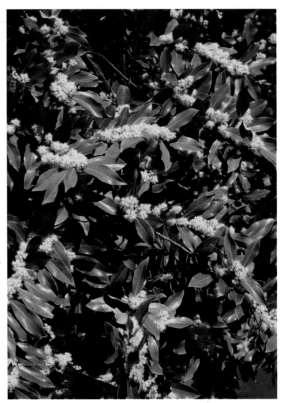

BOTANICAL NAME: *Prunus cerasifera 'Atropurpurea'*
COMMON NAME: **PURPLE LEAF PLUM**
USDA ZONES: 6, 7, 8, 9
ORIGIN: Asia
FORM: Woody deciduous broadleaf tree, up to 25' tall
DESCRIPTION: Copper-red leaves turning deep purple to greenish-bronze, 1-1/2" to 3" long, elliptic in shape
FLOWER COLOR: Pink, white, 1" wide, in clusters, blooms in spring, matures into plums
EXPOSURE: Full sun
WATER: Moderate
GROWTH RATE: Fast
CHARACTERISTICS: Will tolerate some drought and alkaline soils. Susceptible to aphids, scale, spider mites, and borers in the trunk at the crown. Prune in winter to shape. Fruit is edible, but can be messy if planted in the wrong place such as walkways and sidewalks.
USES: Fruit, small shade tree, leaf color, flowering tree, background, and street tree.

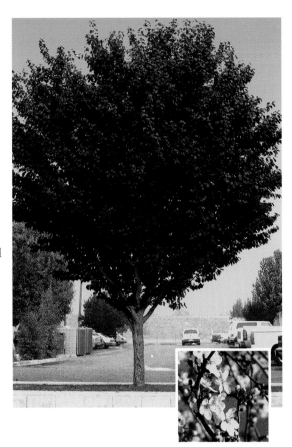

BOTANICAL NAME: *Pyrus calleryana*
COMMON NAME: ORNAMENTAL PEAR
USDA ZONES: 6, 7, 8
ORIGIN: China
FORM: Woody deciduous upright broadleaf tree, up to 25' tall
DESCRIPTION: Dark green leaves, 1-1/2" to 3" long, oval in shape, undulate margins, branches are very erect
FLOWER COLOR: White, 1" wide, in clusters, blooms in late winter
EXPOSURE: Full sun
WATER: Moderate
GROWTH RATE: Fast when young, then slows down
CHARACTERISTICS: Branches characteristically sweep up vertically with almost no lateral growth. Prune out inner branches to open-up. Susceptible to aphids and fireblight. Gophers sometimes like to gnaw on the crown and roots.
USES: Early flowering tree, lawn tree, narrow area, patio tree, and accent.

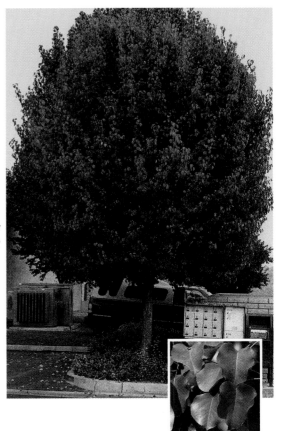

BOTANICAL NAME: *Pyrus kawakamii*
COMMON NAME: EVERGREEN PEAR
USDA ZONES: 9, 10
ORIGIN: Japan, Taiwan
FORM: Woody evergreen or deciduous broadleaf tree, up to 30' tall
DESCRIPTION: Light green glossy leaves turning red, orange and brown in fall, leathery texture, 3" to 4" long by 3" wide, oval in shape, undulate and serrate margins, pointed at the tip
FLOWER COLOR: White, 1" wide, in clusters, blooms in late winter before leaves appear
EXPOSURE: Full sun, partial shade
WATER: Moderate
GROWTH RATE: Fast when young, then slows down
CHARACTERISTICS: Will keep its leaves except where winters are cold. Good fall colors. Susceptible to aphids and fireblight. Prune to shape when young, however, heavy pruning will prevent flowering. Stake for support. Flower petals are very light and will scatter in the wind.
USES: Early flowering tree, street tree, espalier, patio, lawn tree, screen, container, and accent.

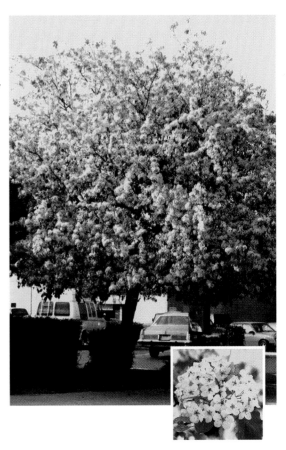

BOTANICAL NAME: *Rhus lancea*
COMMON NAME: **AFRICAN SUMAC**
USDA ZONES: 8
ORIGIN: South Africa
FORM: Woody evergreen broadleaf tree, up to 25' tall
DESCRIPTION: Dark green leaves, 4" to 5" long, "willow like," compound divided into 3 leaflets, 4" to 5" long
FLOWER COLOR: Inconspicuous, matures into fruit
EXPOSURE: Full sun
WATER: Moderate or infrequent once established
GROWTH RATE: Slow
CHARACTERISTICS: Graceful weeping branches. Fruit can be messy. Tree appearance is open and airy. Will tolerate high summer heat. Bark rough and red. Grows as a single or multi-stemmed tree.
USES: Screen, background, large shrub, small tree, and infrequent irrigated area.

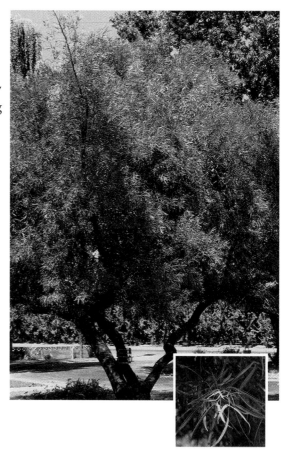

BOTANICAL NAME: *Sapium sebiferum*
COMMON NAME: **CHINESE TALLOW**
USDA ZONES: 4, 5, 6, 7, 8, 9
ORIGIN: China
FORM: Woody deciduous broadleaf tree, up to 40' tall
DESCRIPTION: Light green leaves turning crimson-red to yellow in fall, 3" long, oval in shape, pointed at the tip, distinctive midrib
FLOWER COLOR: Yellow, on 4" long spike, not showy, blooms in late spring
EXPOSURE: Full sun
WATER: Moderate and regular
GROWTH RATE: Moderate to fast
CHARACTERISTICS: Fantastic fall color. Best time to select trees is in the fall so you can see what the fall colors will be like because they will vary from tree to tree. An all around excellent tree that tolerates heat, some drought, and some wind. Prefers slightly acidic soils. Resistant to oak root fungus. Prune to shape when young. Oily seeds when crushed. Seeds can be a mild problem.
USES: Street tree, fall color, light shade tree, accent, and background.

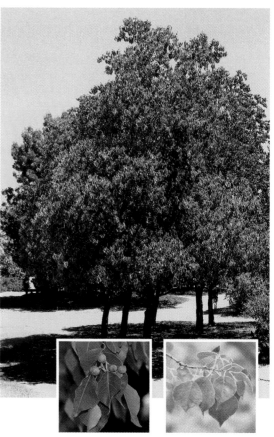

BOTANICAL NAME: *Sequoia sempervirens*
COMMON NAME: **COASTAL REDWOOD**
USDA ZONES: 6, 7, 8, 9
ORIGIN: Coastal ranges of Oregon and California.
FORM: Woody evergreen coniferous tree, 60' to 90' tall, and much taller in their native habitat
DESCRIPTION: Light green needles turning medium to dark green with age, 1/4" to 1", flat, in rows, feather-like
FLOWER COLOR: Inconspicuous
EXPOSURE: Full sun, partional shade
WATER: Moderate and regular
GROWTH RATE: Fast, 2' to 6' a year
CHARACTERISTICS: Distinct conical growth habit. Will tolerate modern irrigation systems. Prefers coastal humidity but will grow in drier inland climates. Likes acidic soils. Resistant to oak fungus and termites. Not bothered by many pests.
USES: Woodsy setting, group, background, park, open space, timber (lumber), native setting and wide median.

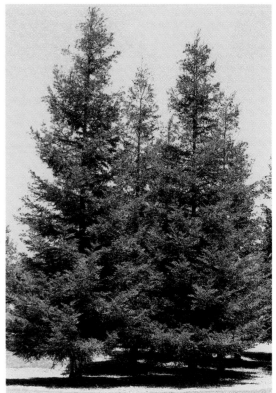

BOTANICAL NAME: *Umbellularia californica*
COMMON NAME: **CALIFORNIA BAY, LAUREL TREE**
USDA ZONES: 7
ORIGIN: Oregon, California coastal range and the lower elevations of the Sierra Nevada mountain range.
FORM: Woody evergreen broadleaf tree or large shrub, up to 25' tall, and taller in its native environment
DESCRIPTION: Medium yellow-green glossy leaves, 2" to 5" long by 1/2" to 1-1/2" wide, lanceolate in shape, light green midrib, leaves aromatic when crushed
FLOWER COLOR: Yellow, small, blooms in spring
EXPOSURE: Full sun to shade
WATER: Moderate and regular
GROWTH RATE: Slow to moderate, about 1' a year
CHARACTERISTICS: Good as a shrub or prune into a tree. Tolerates dry conditions or wet soils. Sometimes hard to find in nurseries. Check with California native plant growers.
USES: Understory plant, screen, background, small tree, California native planting, patio tree, and cooking (leaves).

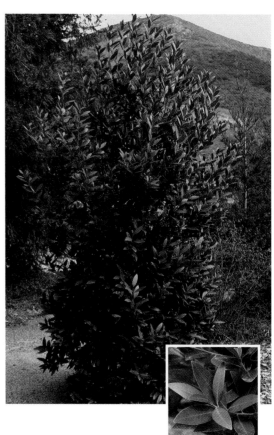

■ BOTANICAL NAME: *Ajuga reptans 'Bronze'*
   COMMON NAME: **BRONZE AJUGA**
   SUNSET ZONES: 3, 4, 5, 6, 7, 8
   ORIGIN: Europe
   FORM: Herbaceous perennial trailing ground cover, up to 12" tall
   DESCRIPTION: Dark green leaves tinged with bronze, 2" to 3" long
   FLOWER COLOR: Blue, 4" to 5" tall, attached to short spikes, blooms from spring to summer
   EXPOSURE: Full sun to partial shade
   WATER: Moderate and regular
   GROWTH RATE: Moderate to fast
   CHARACTERISTICS: Low growing ground cover spreading by runners. Mow spent blooms. Provide good drainage. Plant 6" to 12" apart. Old plants can get ratty and are subject to fungus in areas of poor drainage or air circulation. Several new varieties available. Watch for whiteflies.Will get into lawn so keep barrier between them. Good near contrasting shrubs. Doesn't take foot traffic.
   USES: Flowering ground cover for small confined area or mass planting in large planter.

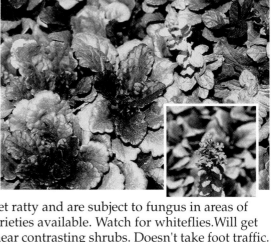

■ BOTANICAL NAME: *Dichondra micrantha (repens or carolinensis)*
   COMMON NAME: **DICHONDRA**
   SUNSET ZONES: 9
   ORIGIN: Texas, New Mexico, Japan, West Indies
   FORM: Herbaceous evergreen ground cover or lawn substitute, 1" to 2" tall, taller in partial shade
   DESCRIPTION: Medium green leaves, 1/2" wide, round in shape, "mouse ear" or miniature "lily pad" looking
   FLOWER COLOR: Inconspicuous
   EXPOSURE: Full sun to partial shade
   WATER: Moderate to high and regular
   GROWTH RATE: Moderate to fast
   CHARACTERISTICS: Tolerates some foot traffic, alkaline soils, heat and semi-shady areas. Best results from seed or closely spaced plugs. Susceptible to flea beetle. Look for browning of the leaves and linear chewing marks on leaves or stems. Spray immediately to control. Fertilize lightly and often (once a month). Considered a moderate to high maintenance ground cover.
   USES: Lawn substitute if foot traffic is infrequent. Ground cover for large or small areas. Between rocks or stones.

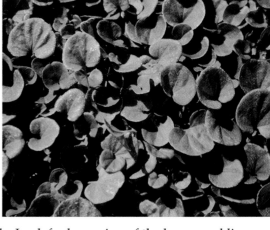

■ BOTANICAL NAME: *Ficus pumila (repens)*
   COMMON NAME: **CREEPING FIG**
   SUNSET ZONES: 9, 10
   ORIGIN: Australia, China, Japan
   FORM: Woody evergreen trailing vine, 15' long or longer
   DESCRIPTION: Light to dark green leaves, young foilage 1" long, heart-shaped, older vigorous foilage 3" long by 1-1/2" wide, oblong in shape
   FLOWER COLOR: Inconspicuous, matures into fruit
   EXPOSURE: Full sun to shade
   WATER: Moderate
   GROWTH RATE: Slow to moderate at first, fast thereafter
   CHARACTERISTICS: Will attach itself to masonry, wood, and metal. Tolerates severe pruning. Prune to control growth and keep full and compact. Can get scale, mealybug, whitefly and thrip.
   USES: Climbing vine for any type of surface on fence or retaining wall, container, house plant, shady area, and ground cover. Can be used on the side of a house, but be sure to keep it trimmed regularly. Will grow in vents, cracks, and eves.

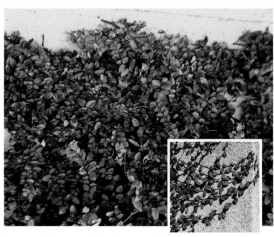

BOTANICAL NAME: *Hedera helix*
COMMON NAME: ENGLISH IVY
SUNSET ZONES: 5, 6, 7, 8, 9, 10
ORIGIN: Europe
FORM: Evergreen broadleaf vine or ground cover, up to 12' long
DESCRIPTION: Dark green leaves, leathery texture, 2" to 4" long, simple with 3 to 5 lobes on margins
FLOWER COLOR: Inconspicuous, in umbels
EXPOSURE: Full sun to shady conditions
WATER: Medium
GROWTH RATE: Rapid
CHARACTERISTICS: Mow ivy on an annual basis to rejuvenate. Prune anytime. Best if contained inside a mow strip. Somewhat invasive and will cling to almost anything. Will not tolerate foot traffic. Very shade tolerant. A playground for snails and slugs.
USES: Ground cover, erosion control, bank cover, fence or wall covering, and indoor container plant.

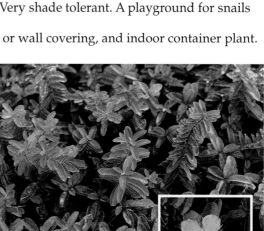

BOTANICAL NAME: *Hypericum calycinum*
COMMON NAME: AARON'S BEARD, HYPERICUM
SUNSET ZONES: 5, 6, 7, 8, 9
ORIGIN: Southeastern Europe
FORM: Evergreen tall ground cover, up to 1' tall
DESCRIPTION: Dark to medium green leaves (depends on the location), 4" long, oblong in shape
FLOWER COLOR: Bright yellow, 2" to 3" wide, yellow stamens, red anthers, blooms in summer
EXPOSURE: Full sun to shade
WATER: Moderate
GROWTH RATE: Moderate to fast, depending on location
CHARACTERISTICS: Tough, excellent ground cover. Spreads by rhizomes. Trampled or dead spots will fill back rather quickly if ground is not compacted. Good competitor, will choke out weeds (said to have allelopathic properties). Susceptible to red spider mite in shady areas. Mow with lawn mower about once a year or when it gets a little rangy looking. Can spread from its area if not bordered with curbing.
USES: Ground cover, bank stabilizer, erosion control, flower, accent, and filler. Good near water.

BOTANICAL NAME: *Mazus reptans*
COMMON NAME: MAZUS
SUNSET ZONE: 6
ORIGIN: Himalayas
FORM: Herbaceous perennial trailing ground cover, 1" to 2" tall
DESCRIPTION: Bright green leaves, 1" long, narrow in shape, lightly serrate margins
FLOWER COLOR: Bluish-purple with white and yellow inflections, 1" wide, in clusters, blooms in late spring
EXPOSURE: Full sun to light shade
WATER: Moderate and regular
GROWTH RATE: Moderate
CHARACTERISTICS: Likes fertile, moist soils. Spreads by rooting stems.
USES: Flowering ground cover, lawn substitute in infrequent foot traffic area, and rock garden.

BOTANICAL NAME: *Pachysandra terminalis*
COMMON NAME: **JAPANESE SPURGE**
SUNSET ZONES: 4, 5, 6, 7, 8
ORIGIN: Japan
FORM: Herbaceous evergreen low growing ground cover, up to 12" tall
DESCRIPTION: Dark green leaves in shade, yellowing in full sun, 2" to 4" long, diamond-shaped, attached to erect stems
FLOWER COLOR: Inconspicuous, greenish-white spikes, small, fragrant, blooms in summer, matures into fruit
EXPOSURE: Deep shade to partial sun
WATER: High until established, moderate thereafter
GROWTH RATE: Slow to moderate
CHARACTERISTICS: Spreads by runners, but is not aggressive. Transplants easily. Fertilize in spring with a complete fertilizer. Pruning is not necessary. Variegated varieties available. Leaves turn yellow in full sun. Whitish fruit in late summer. Plant 6" to 12" apart. Acidic soil is preferred. Flowers fragrant.
USES: Parkway strip, planter, rock garden, and shady area. Good ground cover under trees or as a transition between walkway and lawn area.

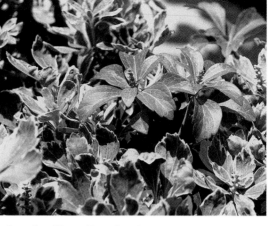

BOTANICAL NAME: *Potentilla verna (tabernaemontanii)*
COMMON NAME: **SPRING CINQUEFOIL**
SUNSET ZONES: 2, 3, 4, 5, 6, 7
ORIGIN: Europe, Asia
FORM: Herbaceous evergreen perennial ground cover, 2" to 6" tall and spreading
DESCRIPTION: Medium to dark green leaves, 1/2" to 1" wide, palmately lobed with serrate margins
FLOWER COLOR: Bright yellow, 1/4" to 3/4" wide, blooms in spring and summer
EXPOSURE: Full sun to partial shade in hot areas
WATER: Moderate and regular
GROWTH RATE: Fast
CHARACTERISTICS: Tolerates coastal conditions, periods of high moisture, occasional mowing and some foot traffic. Susceptible to snails and slugs. Can turn brown during cold winters.
USES: Flowering ground cover, shady area, foreground planting, bank, planter, between stepping stones, and lawn substitue in areas of little foot traffic.

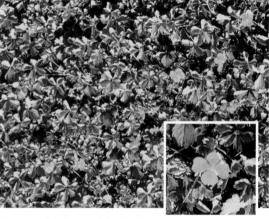

BOTANICAL NAME: *Sagina subulata*
COMMON NAME: **IRISH MOSS**
SUNSET ZONES: 5
ORIGIN: Spain to Northern Russia
FORM: Herbaceous evergreen perennial ground cover, 1" to 4" tall
DESCRIPTION: Dark-green leaves, 1/4" long, moss-like, slender in shape, dense
FLOWER COLOR: White, 1" long, blooms in spring
EXPOSURE: Full sun to partial shade
WATER: Moderate and regular (keep moist)
GROWTH RATE: Moderate to fast
CHARACTERISTICS: Forms a dense low growing mat. Plant on 6" centers for quicker fill-in. Will hump or bunch up as it matures. Cut out narrow strips to keep flat. Will tolerate some light foot traffic, full sun, coastal conditions, and cold temperatures. Will not tolerate deep shade.
USES: Low growing ground cover, good between stepping stones or rocks, border, oriental or woodsy setting.

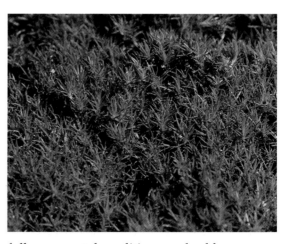

BOTANICAL NAME: *Sedum morganianum*
COMMON NAME: **DONKEY TAIL, BURRO TAIL**
SUNSET ZONES: 10, house plant anywhere
ORIGIN: Central America to Peru
FORM: Herbaceous perennial trailing succulent,
3' to 4' long
DESCRIPTION: Gray-green leaves, 1/2" long, plump, fleshy
(resembles a thick braided rope), bunched on
long pendulous stems
FLOWER COLOR: Pink to deep red, 1/2" long, rare, blooms in
spring
EXPOSURE: Partial shade
WATER: Moderate and regular
GROWTH RATE: Slow to moderate
CHARACTERISTICS: Easily propagated from stem and leaf cuttings.
Protect from the wind. Will grow in poor soils. Fertilize several times during warmer months.
USES: Small scale ground cover, rock and dish gardens, and near pool. Most widely used as a
hanging basket or allowed to cascade over a wall, fence or bank.

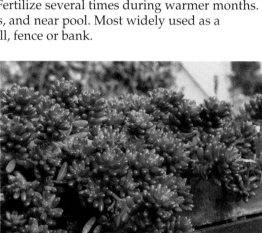

BOTANICAL NAME: *Sedum rubrotinctum (guatemalense)*
COMMON NAME: **PORK AND BEANS**
SUNSET ZONES: 8
ORIGIN: Hybrid
FORM: Herbaceous perennial sprawling succulent,
6" to 8" tall
DESCRIPTION: Medium green leaves with reddish tips
turning almost entirely red in full sun,
3/4" long, round in shape
FLOWER COLOR: Reddish-yellow, 1/2" wide, blooms in spring
EXPOSURE: Full sun to partial shade
WATER: Moderate and regular
GROWTH RATE: Moderate
CHARACTERISTICS: Easily propagated by leaf cuttings. Will not
tolerate foot traffic or over watering.
Relatively maintenance free. Prune occasionally if it gets rangy looking.
USES: Small scale ground cover, planter, border, near pool, semi-shady area, and rock or dish garden.

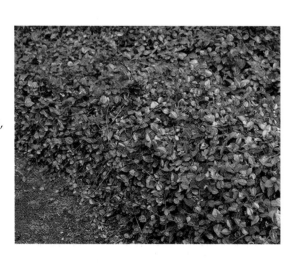

BOTANICAL NAME: *Trachelospermum asiaticum*
COMMON NAME: **ASIAN JASMINE**
SUNSET ZONES: 9
ORIGIN: China, Japan
FORM: Evergreen twining sprawling vine or ground
cover, up to 15' long
DESCRIPTION: Dark green dull leaves, 1" long, oval in shape,
attached to wiry stems
FLOWER COLOR: White to pale yellow, 3/4" wide, in clusters,
fragrant, blooms in late spring
EXPOSURE: Full sun to partial shade in hot areas
WATER: Moderate and regular
GROWTH RATE: Moderate to slow
CHARACTERISTICS: Hardier than most other Jasmine varieties.
Not a vigorous grower. Plant on 10" to 12"
centers for faster cover.
USES: Ground cover, low filler, good light vine, pillar, and espalier. Cut flower for fragrance.

BOTANICAL NAME: *Alcea (Althaea) rosea*
COMMON NAME: HOLLYHOCK
USDA ZONES: 4, all if used as an annual
ORIGIN: Asia Minor
FORM: Biennial (used as an annual), up to 9' tall
DESCRIPTION: Green leaves, large, rough texture, large, round or heart-shaped, with 3, 5 or 7 lobes, main stem is usually hairy
FLOWER COLOR: Pink, purple, yellow, white, red, apricot, 2" to 4" wide, on tall stock, blooms in summer
EXPOSURE: Full sun
WATER: Moderate and regular
GROWTH RATE: Moderate
CHARACTERISTICS: Biennial forms should be planted in the fall. Annual type will bloom the first summer if started in early spring. An old-fashioned flower. Was very popular many years ago. Watch for snails and slugs and remove rust (fungus) infected plants. Plant in rich composted soils of good drainage for best results.
USES: Seasonal color for tall border, planter, container, mass planting in rows or along a fence or house, in the garden on the north side, and near evergreens.

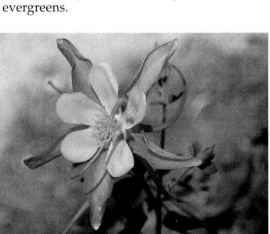

BOTANICAL NAME: *Aquilegia spp.*
COMMON NAME: COLUMBINE
USDA ZONES: 2, 3, 4, 5, 6, 7, 8, 9
ORIGIN: Japan, North America, Hybrid
FORM: Short-lived perennial, delicate, up to 4' tall
DESCRIPTION: Green leaves, 1/2" to 1-1/2" wide, lobed margins, durable, exquisite
FLOWER COLOR: Deep blue, purple and yellow or other combinations such as white, red, violet, 3" wide, blooms from spring to early summer
EXPOSURE: Full sun to partial or filtered shade
WATER: Moderate and regular
GROWTH RATE: Moderate
CHARACTERISTICS: Sow seeds in spring or early summer, transplant if desired by fall. Protect transplants from the sun and wind. Most columbines can also be propagated by root divisions in the fall. Columbines are affected by several insect and fungal disorders. Does best in well drained amended soil. Cut back old stems for additional blooms. Attracts humming birds.
USES: Seasonal color, planter, container, mass planting, rock garden, along fence, and cut garden.

BOTANICAL NAME: *Begonia X semperflorens-cultorum*
COMMON NAME: WAX OR BEDDING BEGONIA
USDA ZONES: 9, used as an annual
ORIGIN: Hybrid
FORM: Herbaceous perennial, 4" to 3' tall and as wide
DESCRIPTION: Bright green to bronzy-red waxy and ` glossy leaves, 2" to 4" long
FLOWER COLOR: Rosy red, white, pink, 1"wide, blooms from spring to fall
EXPOSURE: Partial shade to shade, full sun in mild areas
WATER: Moderate and regular
GROWTH RATE: Moderate to fast
CHARACTERISTICS: Succulent root system. Mostly used as an annual. Propagates easily from leaf and stem cuttings. Susceptible to snails and slugs, aphids, mites, thrip, whitefly, oak root fungus, powdery mildew, and leaf spot. Grows best in rich, well drained high organic soils. Do not constantly over water.
USES: Seasonal color for border, planter, indoor, mass planting, window planter, and entryway.

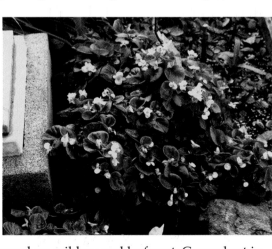

BOTANICAL NAME: *Campanula spp.*
COMMON NAME: **BELLFLOWER**
USDA ZONES: 5, used as an annual
ORIGIN: Mediterranean area
FORM: Annual, biennial or perennial herbs, 6" to 6' tall
DESCRIPTION: Green leaves, smooth texture, 1" to 8" long, oval to heart-shaped, extremely variable, undulate margins
FLOWER COLOR: Blue, lavender, violet, purple, white, 1/2" to 2" wide by 1" long, blooms from spring to fall
EXPOSURE: Full sun in mild areas, partial shade in others
WATER: Moderate and regular
GROWTH RATE: Slow to fast, check on species
CHARACTERISTICS: Sow seeds in spring (transplant if desired) for flowers the next year (perennials and biennials). Divide clumps every 3 to 4 years. Watch for snails and slugs. Many forms available, from trailing or hanging, to upright and erect. A campanula for almost every location in the garden. Flowers bell or wheel-shaped.
USES: Mass plant the lower growing form, perennial border, planter, accent, color, and rock garden.

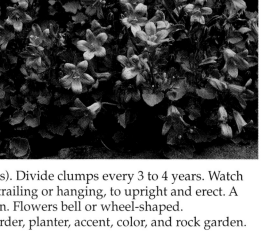

BOTANICAL NAME: *Canna spp.*
COMMON NAME: **CANNA**
USDA ZONES: 2, 3, 4, 5, 6, 7, 8, 9
ORIGIN: West Indies, North and South American tropics
FORM: Herbaceous perennial, 3' to 6' tall
DESCRIPTION: Green to bronzy leaves, 1-1/2' to 4' long by 8" wide, entire margins, looks tropical
FLOWER COLOR: White, ivory, yellow, orange, pink, red, apricot, coral, scarlet, crimson, 3" wide, blooms from summer to fall
EXPOSURE: Full sun
WATER: Moderate to high during flowering
GROWTH RATE: Moderate
CHARACTERISTICS: Flowers on tall spikes and showy. Easily propagated by dividing fleshy, tuberlike roots. Many hybrids available. Easily grown in most soils, especially well-amended soils. Frost sensitive, so dig up roots and store in cool dry place until next spring. Cut back in mild winter areas with the roots left in place.
USES: Mass planting, garden color, background, seasonal light screen, near pool, tropical setting, border, and floral arrangement (leaves used, not the flower).

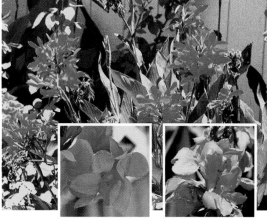

BOTANICAL NAME: *Catharanthus roseus (Vinca rosea)*
COMMON NAME: **PERIWINKLE**
USDA ZONES: 3, 4, 5, 6, 7, 8, 9 10, used as an annual
ORIGIN: Madagascar to India
FORM: Herbaceous perennial, 1' to 2' tall
DESCRIPTION: Green glossy leaves, 1" to 2" long, oblong in shape
FLOWER COLOR: White with pink to red or bluish-pink centers, 1-1/2" wide, blooms late spring to fall
EXPOSURE: Full sun to partial shade
WATER: Moderate and regular
GROWTH RATE: Moderate to fast
CHARACTERISTICS: Good flowering plant in hot arid or humid climates. Simple, but massive flowers and compact. Do not over water. Periwinkle has a long blooming period. Generally from summer to fall and even to Thanksgiving in warmer climates.
USES: Mass planting, border, planter, container, accent, color, rock garden, entryway, path, and transition between sun and shade.

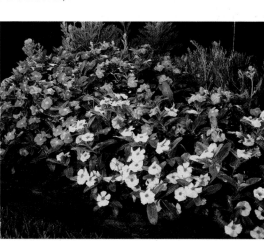

BOTANICAL NAME: *Cymbidium hybridus*
COMMON NAME: **ORCHID**
USDA ZONES: 10, 11
ORIGIN: Southeast Asia
FORM: Evergreen perennial, up to 6' tall
DESCRIPTION: Green leaves, 3' to 4' long by 1" to 3" wide (resembles giant "grass blade"), long and narrow in shape
FLOWER COLOR: Yellow, green, white, pink, bronze with yellow and deep red markings, attached to 2' long spikes, blooms in spring
EXPOSURE: Full sun in mild areas, partial shade in others
WATER: Moderate and regular
GROWTH RATE: Slow
CHARACTERISTICS: Classic flower of Hawaiian Islands. Fertilize with a high nitrogen complete fertilizer during the first six months of the year, low nitrogen fertilizer during the last six months of the year. Best grown in containers where crowded roots produce better blooms. Soil mix should contain peat moss, sand, and forest humus.
USES: Mostly grown for its flowers in arrangements, Hawaiian flower necklace (lei), and novelty.

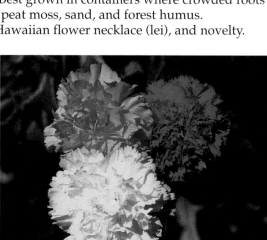

BOTANICAL NAME: *Dianthus carophyllus*
COMMON NAME: **CARNATION**
USDA ZONES: 5, used as an annual
ORIGIN: Central and Eastern China
FORM: Semi-herbaceous annual, biennial or short lived perennial, up to 4' tall
DESCRIPTION: Gray basal leaves, 1" long by 1/2" wide, narrow in shape, hairy margins
FLOWER COLOR: Purple, yellow, variegated, hybrid colors of white, pink, red, and others, 3" wide, blooms in summer
EXPOSURE: Full sun, afternoon shade
WATER: Moderate
GROWTH RATE: Moderate
CHARACTERISTICS: Tall erect flower that often times needs support. Mass plant for stability. Sow seed in place or reproduce by rooting basal stem cuttings. Remove spent flowers and stalks to prolong blooming period. Flowers are not very fragrant if at all. Wilt disease such as stem rot and anthracnose can cause problems. Remove diseased plants at once. Keep foliage dry. Can get red spider mites.
USES: Cut flower, garden flower, container, background flower, commercial use, and arrangement.

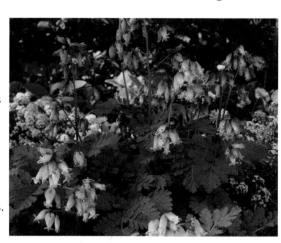

BOTANICAL NAME: *Dicentra spp.*
COMMON NAME: **BLEEDING HEART**
USDA ZONES: 3, 4, 5, 6, 7, 8, 9
ORIGIN: Pacific Coast, Japan, Northeast United States
FORM: Herbacious perennial, 8" to 3' tall
DESCRIPTION: Blue-green or soft green basal leaves (depends on species), dainty, fern-like, parted margins
FLOWER COLOR: Rose-pink to rose, 5/8" long, heart-shaped, spurred petals, blooms in summer
EXPOSURE: Shade to partial shade
WATER: Moderate
GROWTH RATE: Moderate
CHARACTERISTICS: Needs well-drained soil, rich with amendments. Has a dormant period. Propagate by division.
USES: Native planting, shady area, planter, accent, hillside, near rocks, and container.

BOTANICAL NAME: *Eschscholzia californica*
COMMON NAME: CALIFORNIA POPPY
USDA ZONES: 9, 10, 11, annual anywhere
ORIGIN: California
FORM: Herbaceous perennial or annual, up to 2' tall
DESCRIPTION: Bluish-green leaves, 4" to 6" long, almost fern-like, finely lobed or parted margins
FLOWER COLOR: Orange, yellow, 3/4" to 2-1/4" wide, attached to tall stalks, blooms from spring to summer
EXPOSURE: Full sun
WATER: Moderate
GROWTH RATE: Moderate
CHARACTERISTICS: State flower of California. Reseeds easily. Looks best from a distance. Gophers eat the roots. Will tolerate dry conditions but blooms best with regular water. Does not transplant well. Sow seed in the fall or plant from pony packs.
USES: Native planting, accent, hillside, bank cover, roadway, near rocks, cut flower, and container.

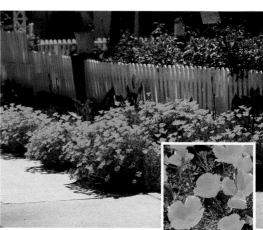
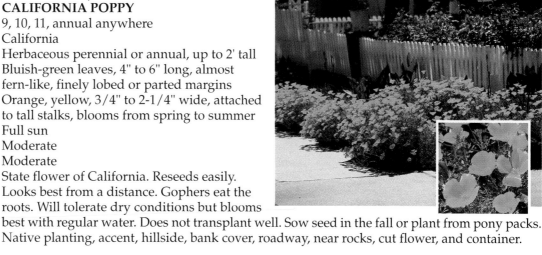

BOTANICAL NAME: *Gladiolus spp.*
COMMON NAME: GLADIOLUS
USDA ZONES: 6, 7, 8, 9
ORIGIN: Tropical Africa, Mediterranean area, Asia
FORM: Herbaceous perennial, up to 5' tall, stout
DESCRIPTION: Green basal leaves, 12" to 18" long by 1" wide, sword-like
FLOWER COLOR: Orange, yellow, red, purple, white, salmon, rose, lavender, 1-1/2' to 2-1/2' long by 1/2" to 1" wide, attached to tall stalks, blooms in spring, summer or fall
EXPOSURE: Full sun
WATER: Moderate and regular
GROWTH RATE: Moderate
CHARACTERISTICS: Grow from a corm (bulb-like). Best in well-prepared soil with amendments. Plant corms four times as deep as the corm is tall (usually 3" to 4" deep). Re-cut flower stem under water for longer lasting arrangements. In mild areas leave corms in ground all year. In cold climates, dig up corms after first frost, let dry and store on trays or ventilated bags and store in a cool place, but above freezing. Watch for thrips they can discolor the flowers. Gladiolus can get fungal, bacterial and viral disorders including dry rot, leaf blight, mosaic and white break. Spray or dust accordingly.
USES: Cut flower, wedding and funeral flowers, accent, garden, near rocks, background border, and container.

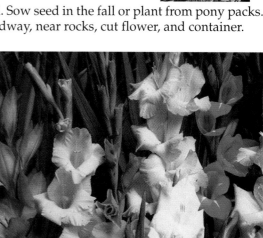

BOTANICAL NAME: *Hemerocallis spp.*
COMMON NAME: DAYLILY
USDA ZONES: 3, 4, 5, 6, 7, 8, 9
ORIGIN: Japan, Eastern Asia
FORM: Semi-herbaceous perennial, up to 6' tall
DESCRIPTION: Medium green basal leaves, 1' to 1-1/2' long by 1" wide, arching and sword-like, some with undulate margins, some are deciduous
FLOWER COLOR: Orange, yellow, red, white, pink, purple, apricot, bicolor, 3-1/2" wide by 3" to 5" long, tubular in shape, blooms from spring to fall
EXPOSURE: Full sun to light shade best
WATER: Moderate and regular
GROWTH RATE: Slow to moderate
CHARACTERISTICS: In mild winter areas daylilies can bloom almost year round. Remove dead leaves and flower stalks. Cut back entire plant if they get ratty looking in late winter. Spray to control aphids. Will grow in many types of soil.
USES: Cut flower, accent, garden, near rocks, background border, container, near pool, and entryway.

BOTANICAL NAME: *Iris spp.*
COMMON NAME: **BEARDED IRIS**
USDA ZONES: 2, 3, 4, 5, 6, 7, 8, 9, 10, 11
ORIGIN: Hybrid
FORM: Herbaceous, rhizominous perennial, 1' to 4' tall
DESCRIPTION: Medium green basal leaves, 1' to 2' long by 1" wide, strap-shaped, flat, pointed at the tip
FLOWER COLOR: Blue, white, red, yellow, 1" to 3" long (varies with species), attached to stalks, blooms in spring
EXPOSURE: Full sun to partial shade
WATER: Moderate
GROWTH RATE: Fast
CHARACTERISTICS: Grows from rhizomes. Stake flower stalks in windy areas. Remove dead flower stalks and leaves. Plant between spring and fall. Likes well-drained soils.
USES: Cut flower, seasonal border, planter, container, accent, near water, and novelty.

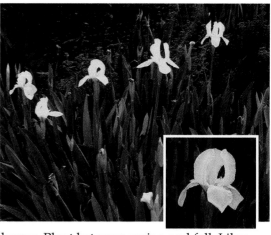

BOTANICAL NAME: *Narcissus spp.*
COMMON NAME: **DAFFODIL**
USDA ZONES: 3, 4, 5, 6, 7, 8
ORIGIN: Europe, North Africa
FORM: Herbaceous perennial bulbs, up to 18" tall
DESCRIPTION: Dark green leaves, 18" long (variable), strap shaped or semi-triangular in shape
FLOWER COLOR: Mostly yellow and white, some orange, red, cream, pink, blooms in spring
EXPOSURE: Full sun
WATER: Moderate
GROWTH RATE: Moderate
CHARACTERISTICS: Plant bulbs in the fall 4" to 6" deep and at least 8" apart. Bulbs multiply readily. Let foliage die back naturally. This will help insure good blooms for next year. Different flower shapes are available.
USES: Seasonal color, cut flower, planter, container, native planting, near rocks, and border.

BOTANICAL NAME: *Paeonia hybridus*
COMMON NAME: **PEONY**
USDA ZONES: 2, 3, 4, 5, 6, 7, 8
ORIGIN: Hybrid
FORM: Herbaceous perennial tubers, 2' to 4' tall
DESCRIPTION: Deep green leaves, 3" to 10" long by 2" to 6" wide, neatly divided margins
FLOWER COLOR: White, cream, red, pink, 3" to 4" wide, blooms in spring
EXPOSURE: Full sun
WATER: Moderate
GROWTH RATE: Moderate
CHARACTERISTICS: Plants need a good winter chill to really produce quality flowers. Plant in early fall preparing the soil 18" to 2' deep and add some humus. Plant about 1-1/2" to 2" deep with the eyes of the tubers upward. Needs average fertilizer, and flowers may need staking. Divide in fall if necessary.
USES: Excellent cut flower, perennial border, planter, and container.

BOTANICAL NAME: *Ranunculus asiaticus*
COMMON NAME: **RANUNCULUS**
USDA ZONES: All zones if used as an annual
ORIGIN: Europe, Asia
FORM: Herbaceous perennial tubers, 18" to 2' tall
DESCRIPTION: Medium green leaves, 1" to 2" wide, divided with 3 lobes, cleft margins
FLOWER COLOR: White, cream, yellow, orange, red, pink, 3" to 5" wide, blooms in spring
EXPOSURE: Full sun
WATER: Moderate
GROWTH RATE: Moderate
CHARACTERISTICS: Plant in the fall 2" deep or 1/2" to 1" deep in heavy soils with the prongs downward. Keep moist, but do not over water. Cover with netting if birds are a problem. Let plant die completely down before digging it up for storage.
USES: Perennial border, planter, cut flower, and mass planting, especially with other perennials.

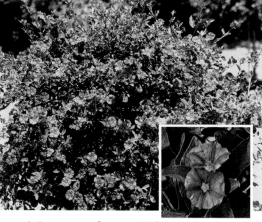

BOTANICAL NAME: *Solanum rantonnetii (lycianthes rantonnei)*
COMMON NAME: **BLUE SOLANUM,**
BLUE POTATO BUSH
USDA ZONES: 9
ORIGIN: Paraguay, Argentina
FORM: Woody evergreen to semi-deciduous shrub or vining ground cover, up to 8' tall by 15' long
DESCRIPTION: Bright green leaves, 4" long, oval in shape, leaves fall-off in cold weather
FLOWER COLOR: Violet to dark blue with yellow center, 1" wide, blooms during warm weather
EXPOSURE: Full sun to partial shade
WATER: Moderate
GROWTH RATE: Fast
CHARACTERISTICS: Prune severely to keep in check or let it sprawl as a vining ground cover. Tolerates heat, and coastal conditions. Can get aphids, scale, and caterpillars. Very long bloomer especially in warm or hot areas. Very informal looking.
USES: Flowering ground cover, filler, espalier, bank cover, and mass planting.

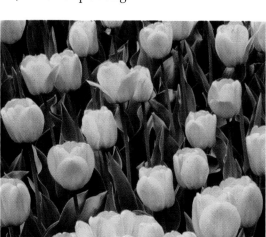

BOTANICAL NAME: *Tulipa spp.*
COMMON NAME: **TULIP**
USDA ZONES: 3, 4, 5, 6, 7, 8, 9
ORIGIN: Hybrid
FORM: Herbaceous perennial bulbs, up to 30" tall
DESCRIPTION: Medium green basal leaves, 6" wide (resembles big "elf ears")
FLOWER COLOR: Red, yellow, white, pink, purple, 4" wide, solid or striped, blooms in late spring
EXPOSURE: Full sun
WATER: Moderate
GROWTH RATE: Moderate
CHARACTERISTICS: Provide afternoon shade in hot areas for longer lasting blooms. Plant in rich well-draining or sandy soil 2-1/2" deeper than the bulb is wide and about 8" apart. Protect from gophers, mice, and aphids. Many varieties available. Best results with good winter chill.
USES: Container, cut flower, planter, perennial garden, mass planting, accent, and spring color.

BOTANICAL NAME: *Verbena spp.*
COMMON NAME: **VERBENA**
USDA ZONES: 2, 3, 4, 5, 6, 7, 8, 9, 10, annual
ORIGIN: North and South America
FORM: Herbaceous perennial short lived ground cover or shrub, up to 18" tall
DESCRIPTION: Green leaves, 2" to 4" wide, mum-like, semi-sparse
FLOWER COLOR: Purple, red, blue, white, rose, lavender, 2" to 3" wide, in clusters, blooms from summer to fall
EXPOSURE: Full sun
WATER: Moderate
GROWTH RATE: Moderate to fast
CHARACTERISTICS: Flowers best in warm to hot climates. Fast growing in the hot summers. Do not over water or the plant will die. Provide good drainage. Often treated as an annual. Can get ratty looking. Cut back bad areas or remove and replant. Cultivated varieties produce vibrant and abundant blooms. Native species are rarely cultivated. They are rather weedy looking with far less attractive blooms. Can get mildew, spider mites and whiteflies.
USES: Flowering ground cover, colorful border, hanging basket, planter, annual, and rock garden.

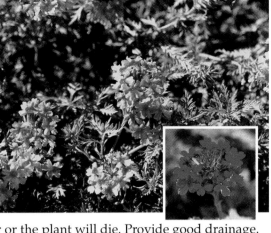

BOTANICAL NAME: *Viola X wittrockiana*
COMMON NAME: **PANSY**
USDA ZONES: 2, 3, 4, 5, 6, 7, 8, 9, 10, annual
ORIGIN: Hybrid
FORM: Herbaceous annual, 4" to 9" tall and as wide
DESCRIPTION: Dark green glossy leaves, 2" to 6" long petioles, oblong in shape, revolute margins
FLOWER COLOR: White, red, purple, yellow, blue, mixed, 2" to 4" wide, blooms from winter to spring
EXPOSURE: Full sun
WATER: Moderate
GROWTH RATE: Slow to moderate
CHARACTERISTICS: Pinch out old blooms to keep plants flowering. Best in cool climates. Will not tolerate hot temperatures. Lightly fertilize every two to three weeks. Can be bothered by snails, slugs, mites and thrips.
USES: Great winter and spring colors, border, planter, container, cut flower, mass planting, near rocks, and understory to larger shrubs.

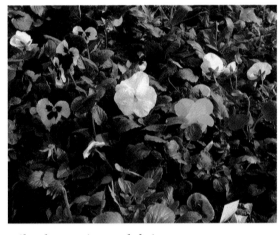

BOTANICAL NAME: *Zantedeschia spp.*
COMMON NAME: **CALLA**
USDA ZONES: 7
ORIGIN: South Africa
FORM: Herbaceous rhizomatous stemless flowering shrub, up to 3' tall
DESCRIPTION: Rich green glossy leaves sometimes with white spots, 18" tall by 10" wide, attached to long stalks, arrow-like undulate margins
FLOWER COLOR: Yellow, white, pink, orange, 5" to 10" long spathe, blooms from spring to summer
EXPOSURE: Full sun, partial shade in hot climates
WATER: Moderate to high
GROWTH RATE: Slow to moderate
CHARACTERISTICS: The color isn't from the flower, rather it is from the spathe. Roots are actually rhizomes. Fertilize lightly after blooming. Can get root rot and other disorders, watch for aphids.
USES: Cut flower, arrangement, understory, semi-shaded area, planter, entryway, bordering a window, near tropical plants, and near rocks.

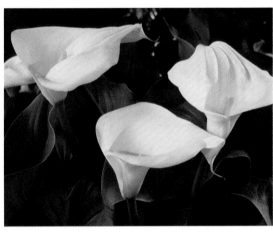

Allergy Producing Plants

Definition

A plant that at some period of time (season) produces significant quantities of pollen (usually wind blown) which causes an allergenic reaction in selective numbers of the populous.

Explanation of Format

In a previous chapter, a classification was established for the two types of pollen. Now we must confine our classification into a definition setting forth the criteria that will determine the plants that are considered to be the allergy producers.

The balance of this chapter is dedicated to exposing these plants and listing certain characteristics including botanical and common name, USDA growing zones, degree of allergenic severity, months of allergenic severity, areas of known plant existence and concentrations, and areas of known allergy relief and partial relief.

Each plant is listed by its **Botanical Name.** However, the **Common Name** is also included for familiarity and laymen identification, and can be crossed referenced in the index. The **USDA Zones** indicate where the allergy producing plants grow according to their cold temperature sensitivity. The USDA Zones generally deal with ornamental plants.

Next is the **Degree of Allergenic Severity.** This categorizes the allergy producing plants into three areas. **High, Moderate** and **Occasional** with "high" causing the worst allergenic reactions in greater numbers of people, followed by "Moderate" which can and do cause allergies but generally in fewer people, and/or cause less of a reaction. Lastly, "occasional" are plants with very short pollen seasons, and/or cause mild allergy reactions in still fewer people.

The last section is an attempt to pinpoint specific geographic areas where the allergy plants **Exist,** where they are most **Concentrated,** and where (if anywhere) there is **Relief** or **Partial Relief** from the allergy producing plant.

I would like to make it very clear that this last section is a guide and should not excite anyone to pack-up and move away from or into any of these areas thinking that their allergy problems will be solved. It is my intent that the reader use this section to better prepare himself/herself for traveling from or into different areas of the United States. An example would be, when you or your family are planning a vacation or trip and would like to be prepared for possible allergy problems. Nothing is worse than to plan a relaxing vacation in an area where you end up in misery because of allergies.

Plant Allergy Maps for the Traveler

If you have allergies and travel, you know the two do not mix. Vacations, business travel, weekend getaways and family visits can take you from the "frying pan and put you into the fire". For this reason plant allergy maps are included with each plant that **Grows Naturally** in the United States. Some allergy producing plants are not native to the United States and grow only in urban and rural areas. These plants are considered "locally common" and have a map showing areas where the plant "can" grow. The shaded areas on each map indicate the areas where the plant might be found growing naturally (native and naturalized plants).

The **Months of Allergenic Severity** are listed below the map and indicate when the plant is pollinating. Pollinating periods can vary depending on weather and regional areas. Midwest and Eastern states generally have later spring and summer seasons, than the West. Altitude also plays an important part in plant pollination. Minor adjustments may need to be considered depending on your specific location.

BOTANICAL NAME: *Artemisia spp.*
COMMON NAME: **SAGEBRUSH, WORMWOOD, MUGWORT**

DEGREE OF ALLERGENIC SEVERITY: High

AREAS OF KNOWN PLANT

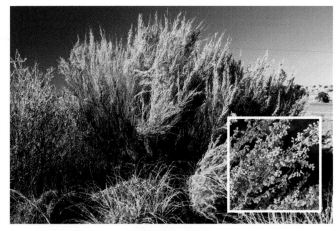

EXISTENCE:
Sagebrush grows in arid mountain slopes, high plains, and woods, often in association with rabbitbrush, saltbrush and black greasewood. Next to ragweed and grasses, sagebrush is the most important cause of allergies in the West. Some artemisia species are used as ornamentals and have escaped into the natural landscape especially from New York to Minnesota.

CONCENTRATIONS:
Sagebrush covers about 100,000,000 acres of land in the West. It is found growing in valleys and foothills, plains of Utah, southern Idaho, Colorado, New Mexico, Arizona, Montana, Wyoming, eastern Washington, including along the Columbia River and tributaries and Eastern Oregon, East of the Sierra Nevada Mountains, Antelope Valley and along the coast in California especially in Monterey and Humbolt Counties. Sagebrush is the most abundant plant in the entire Great Basin. It also can be found in the Mojave desert. Sagebrush generally grows between 2,000 feet to 10,000 feet in elevation on sandy soils.

In the East, sagebrush grows to a lesser extent than in the west, however, it is found in many Midwest and Eastern states including Delaware, New Jersey New York, Pennsylvania (New England states), sparsely in Georgia,

  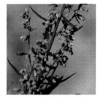

Michigan, Wisconsin, and Minnesota, Kansas, Oklahoma, Arkansas, and Texas. There are many artemisia species.

AREAS OF KNOWN ALLERGY

RELIEF:
West side of the Sierra Nevada Mountains above the chaparral community. Northern Idaho, western Washington and Oregon.

PARTIAL RELIEF:
San Joaquin Valley, California, southern parts of the Gulf States.

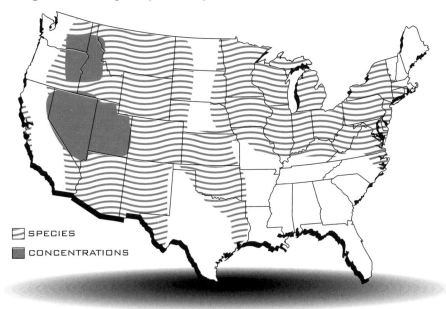

SPECIES
CONCENTRATIONS

MONTHS OF ALLERGENIC SEVERITY

| JAN | FEB | MAR | APR | MAY | JNE | JLY | AUG | SEPT | OCT | NOV | DEC |

BOTANICAL NAME: *Atriplex spp.*
COMMON NAME: **SALTBRUSH**

DEGREE OF ALLERGENIC SEVERITY: Moderate to High

AREAS OF KNOWN PLANT

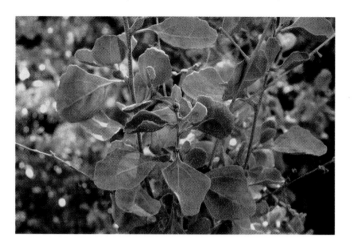

EXISTENCE:
 A widely distributed species of plants from sea level to 7,000 feet. Atriplex likes alkaline soils but will grow in more fertile soils. It can be seen growing in desert or semi-arid conditions.

NATURAL CONCENTRATIONS:
 Saltbrush is one of the most common shrubs of the Great Basin in Nevada. It extends southward into New Mexico and Arizona, the Sonora and Mojave Deserts, and along the Colorado River. In California, throughout Owens Valley, Trucky River near Pyramid Lake, San Francisco area, San Luis Obispo and Los Angeles Counties, San Joaquin Valley, east of the Cascade and Sierra Nevada Mountains to southwestern Montana, Wyoming, Idaho, Texas Panhandle, and Utah. It often grows in association with big sagebrush and creosote brush, especially in the desert areas. An important cause of allergy in the San Francisco Bay area and Arizona.

 In the East, saltbrush grows with less abundance than the West and is reported to be only a minor allergy problem. It is found from New England states into Quebec (St. Lawrence River Gulf, Canada), to Montana, Long Island, New York, Kentucky, Missouri, Kansas, Nebraska, Atlantic and Gulf Coast states, and in salt marshes of Florida.

AREAS OF KNOWN ALLERGY

RELIEF:
 Unknown

PARTIAL RELIEF:
 West of the Cascade Mountains in Oregon and Washington. Above 8,000 feet in elevation. Some parts of the interior eastern states and mid western states away from marshy and sandy soils.

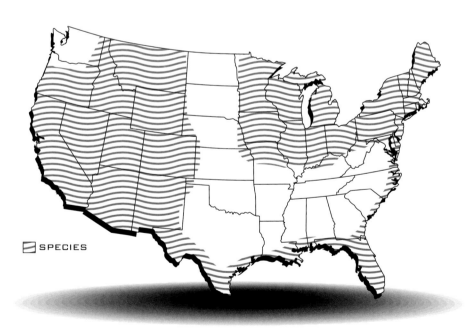

▨ SPECIES

MONTHS OF ALLERGENIC SEVERITY

| JAN | FEB | MAR | APR | MAY | JNE | JLY | AUG | SEPT | OCT | NOV | DEC |

■ BOTANICAL NAME: *Ceanothus spp.*
COMMON NAME   **CEANOTHUS,**
                    NEW JERSEY TEA,
                    SNOWBRUSH
USDA ZONES: 4, 5, 6, 7, 8, 9

DEGREE OF ALLERGENIC SEVERITY: Moderate

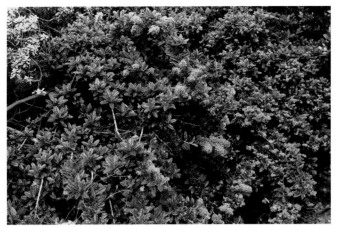

AREAS OF KNOWN PLANT

EXISTENCE:

Ceanothus grows naturally in canyons and shaded slopes in mixed coniferous forests, and scrubby brushy areas usually to 2,300 feet in elevation. It likes light and well-drained soils in sunny locations. Easterly ceanothus grows in dry, open woods (pines), and dry or gravely banks. Ceanothus is also a popular ornamental landscape shrub and is moderately "locally common" within its respected USDA climate zones.

NATURAL CONCENTRATIONS:

Ceanothus is found naturally in California, in burned areas on the eastern slope of the Sierra Nevada Mountains, along interstate 80 and the Donnar Lake area. On the western slope of the Sierra Nevada you can find ceanothus growing from Tulare County (El Capitan), northward to Modoc, Humbolt, and Trinity Counties. Other areas in California include, Yankee Point in Monterey County, San Luis Obispo County, San Diego, Ventura and Orange counties and the Santa Ana Mountains. Throughout the Rocky Mountains, Colorado from 5,500 to 9,000 feet in elevation, high mountain hillsides in northeast Utah and Arizona, extreme western Nevada, southern Oregon and Washington coast through the Cascade Mountains east to Idaho and eastern Montana. They are also found in southwest New Mexico on dry slopes in chaparral and open forest, burned areas of Capitan Mountain and Lincoln National Forest in Central New Mexico, near Salt Creek area to Kingman, Arizona, the Kiibab Plateau and Chiricahua Mountains at the lower edge of the ponderosa pine zone and in the Prescott Forest, South Dakota to Wyoming

In the East, ceanothus is found naturally in Keweenaw County in Michigan, Black Hills in South Dakota, Cape Code in Massachusetts, Cecil County in Maryland, from Maine through Vermont to South Carolina, Georgia to Florida and Alabama extending west to Texas.

AREAS OF KNOWN ALLERGY

RELIEF:

USDA zones 1, 2, Great Basin, Neveda and other desert climates, Florida, and interior plains of Texas.

PARTIAL RELIEF:

Unknown because of its ornamental use.

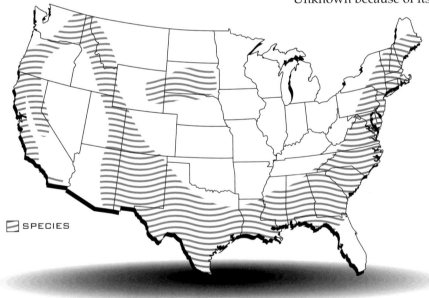

SPECIES

MONTHS OF ALLERGENIC SEVERITY

| JAN | FEB | MAR | APR | MAY | JNE | JLY | AUG | SEPT | OCT | NOV | DEC |

BOTANICAL NAME: *Chrysothamnus spp.*
COMMON NAME: RABBITBRUSH, CHAMISA

DEGREE OF ALLERGENIC SEVERITY: High

AREAS OF KNOWN PLANT

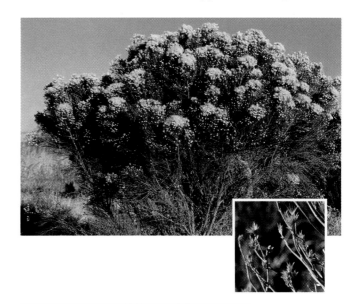

EXISTENCE:
Like most weedy shrubs, the rabbitbrush has spread throughout the West mostly occupying rocky slopes and canyon walls down to open deserts and gravelly washes ranging from 1,000 feet to 10,000 feet in elevation. Rabbitbrush can also be found in areas of over grazing. Rabbitbrush is often found in association with big sagebrush, antelope brush and in juniper and pinyon pine communities up to the borderline of the ponderosa pine communities.

NATURAL CONCENTRATIONS:
The rabbitbrush species is a familiar sight in the Great Basin and outlying areas. In California they can be found growing in the Mojave Desert from Tehachapi to east Inyo and San Bernadino Counties. Also, along the West Coast and coastal mountains on into Oregon and Washington. Other areas include the Santa Rosa Mountains in the Colorado Desert, western Colorado on the alkaline lowlands, plains, foothills and mountains near 6,500 and 8,000 feet in elevation, Utah Desert, Salt Lake Desert, Chihuahua Desert, Little Colorado River, Fault Block Mountains in southeast Oregon and along the John Day River in Oregon, San Juan, Gila, Rio Grande Rivers in New Mexico, mountains in Montana, Yellowstone Park area in Wyoming, and Colorado. Rabbitbrush does not grow in the East.

AREAS OF KNOWN ALLERGY

RELIEF:
East of the Rocky Mountains.

PARTIAL RELIEF:
High elevation above the ponderosa pine forests, parts of the San Joaquin Valley.

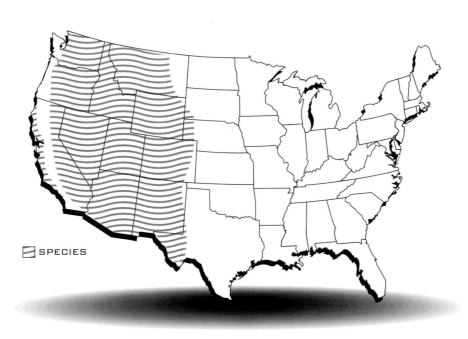

SPECIES

MONTHS OF ALLERGENIC SEVERITY

| JAN | FEB | MAR | APR | MAY | JNE | JLY | AUG | SEPT | OCT | NOV | DEC |

BOTANICAL NAME: *Cortaderia selloana*
COMMON NAME: **PAMPUS GRASS**
USDA ZONES: 5, 6, 7, 8, 9

DEGREE OF ALLERGENIC SEVERITY: Occasional

AREAS OF KNOWN PLANT

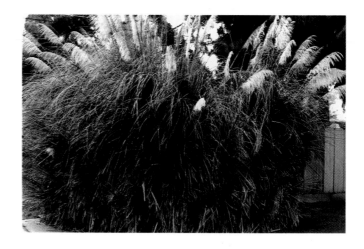

EXISTENCE:
Pampus grass is native to Argentina and has naturalized mostly in California. It is also a semi-popular landscape plant, so consider it to be mildly "locally common" in urban situations. Pampus grass will grow in wet or dry soils in many climatic situations. It has escaped to some areas to become a weed.

NATURAL CONCENTRATIONS:
Pampus grass has naturalized in the coastal bluffs along the California Coast from Ventura to Monterey counties, especially in the Big Sur area and in the San Francisco Bay area up to Humbolt County, near Big Lagoon. Sometimes cultivated as an ornamental in the South which has caused some to escape into the natural landscape.

AREAS OF KNOWN ALLERGY

RELIEF:
USDA zones 1, 2, 3, 4. Natural unpopulated areas of Arizona, New Mexico. The New England States, upper and central Midwest (Kansas north into Canada), and East into the Ohio River Valley.

PARTIAL RELIEF:
Natural unpopulated areas of Washington, Oregon, eastern California. Northern parts of Georgia, inland parts of North and South Carolina, and Virginia.

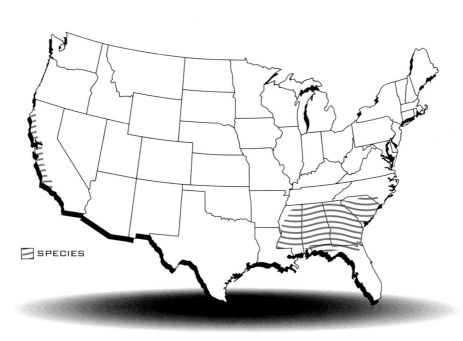

▢ SPECIES

MONTHS OF ALLERGENIC SEVERITY

| JAN | FEB | MAR | APR | MAY | JNE | JLY | AUG | SEPT | OCT | NOV | DEC |

BOTANICAL NAME: *Hymenoclea spp.*
COMMON NAME: BURRO BRUSH

DEGREE OF ALLERGENIC SEVERITY: High

AREAS OF KNOWN PLANT

EXISTENCE:
　　Burro brush grows naturally in sandy washes or drainage areas, alluvial plains and gravelly or rocky slopes below sea level to 5,000 feet in elevation in the West and in Texas.

NATURAL CONCENTRATIONS:
　　Burro brush is found naturally in the southern part of the Great Basin, Chihuahua, Mojave, Colorado, Sonora, and Arizona deserts, also, in the Colorado River area, south of Kingman in Arizona , southwest Utah, the Great Plains and north to Socorro in New Mexico, and southwest Texas. In California burro brush grows in Cuyama Valley, San Luis Obispo, Kern, Riverside, Inyo and San Diego Counties, and in parts of the San Joaquin Valley. Burro brush does not grow east of Texas in any appreciable numbers.

AREAS OF KNOWN ALLERGY

RELIEF:
　　Washington, Idaho, Montana, Wyoming, Oregon, Midwest and Eastern states.

PARTIAL RELIEF:
　　Upper Nevada and Utah, northern California, and central Texas.

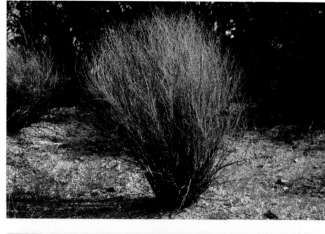

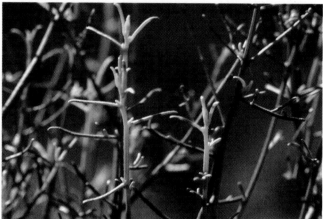

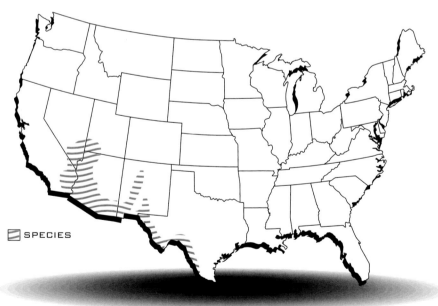

SPECIES

MONTHS OF ALLERGENIC SEVERITY

JAN	FEB	MAR	APR	MAY	JNE	JLY	AUG	SEPT	OCT	NOV	DEC

■ SALSOLA　■ MONOGYRA

BOTANICAL NAME: *Juniperus spp.*
COMMON NAME: **JUNIPER, MEXICAN CEDAR,**
MOUNTAIN CEDAR
USDA ZONES: 3, 4, 5, 6

DEGREE OF ALLERGENIC SEVERITY: Occasional to high

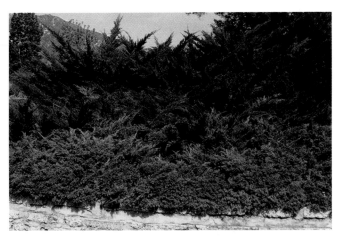

AREAS OF KNOWN PLANT

EXISTENCE:
There are many species of junipers throughout the United States. Some are native and some are introduced. Junipers have been used as an ornamental landscape shrub or small tree for many years. They became popular in the 1950's and 60's as a low maintenance, semi-drought tolerant plant. The juniper species is one of the most planted and widely spread plant in our urban areas and is the most "locally common" allergy shrub in use today. Naturally, junipers grow in mostly rocky soil, dry slopes or plains, in mountainous regions usually in association with pinyon pine, oaks, pastures or in pure stands. Most junipers range from 3,000 and 10,000 feet in elevation. Juniper species differ widely in their allergy producing ability.

NATURAL CONCENTRATIONS:
Junipers are found growing in their native state in eastern Nevada to Utah usually on higher ground or on small mountain slopes. They are also found in the Rocky Mountains and western Colorado, southern Montana, Wyoming, southern Idaho, eastern half of Oregon and Washington, in and around Aldrich Mountains, Flagstaff and San Francisco mountains in Arizona, Albuquerque, Santa Fe, Gallup and northern New Mexico, central

Sierra Nevada Mountains, and other coastal and southern California mountains in California. Also, junipers can be found in the Trans-Pecos in Texas, Alaska to southern Ontario in Canada to Maine and widespread throughout the eastern United States to North Dakota, Wisconson, and Minnesota continuing south through New York, southern Indiana, Mississippi into Florida and Texas. The worst junipers are the mountain Junipers (*Juniperus mexicana, Juniperus sabinoides*) which are found mostly in Texas.

AREAS OF KNOWN ALLERGY

RELIEF:
Unknown.

PARTIAL RELIEF:
Unfortunately, partial relief is going to be hard to find because of juniper's tough adaptability to most United State climates, widespread use as a landscape plant, and large native range and population. South Florida and Louisiana.

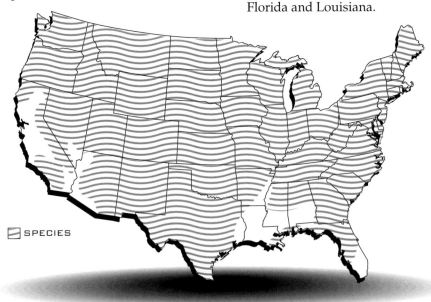

SPECIES

MONTHS OF ALLERGENIC SEVERITY

| JAN | FEB | MAR | APR | MAY | JNE | JLY | AUG | SEPT | OCT | NOV | DEC |

BOTANICAL NAME: *Ligustrum spp.*
COMMON NAME: **PRIVET**
USDA ZONES: 4, 5, 6, 7, 8, 9

DEGREE OF ALLERGENIC SEVERITY: Moderate

AREAS OF KNOWN PLANT

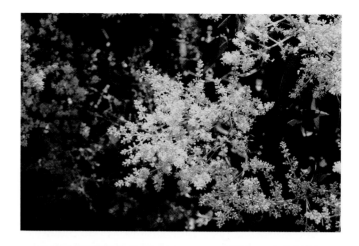

EXISTENCE:
Privets are an introduced plant from Japan and Korea used primarily as an ornamental landscape shrub. Consider them moderately "locally common" in their climate zones. Privet will grow in a multitude of soils and conditions. Most are evergreen but some are deciduous. Privets are established in woodlands and roadsides.

NATURAL CONCENTRATIONS:
Privets are found in cities and towns throughout the United States within its USDA zones 4 to 9. It has been reported to have escaped into the natural landscape in various areas of Colorado, California and the Southwest.
In the East, privets are found in south Maine to North Carolina, southeast Virginia, Ohio, Michigan, and in open woods from New England to Pennsylvania. It is used in the southern states as an ornamental and has, no doubt, moved beyond its ornamental boundaries.

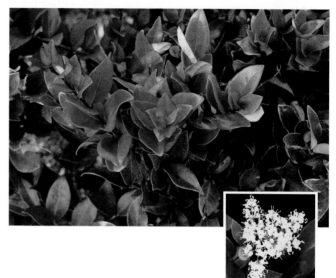

AREAS OF KNOWN ALLERGY

RELIEF:
Possibly USDA zones 1, 2, 3

PARTIAL RELIEF:
Possibly bordering southern Tennessee, northern South Carolina, and Florida.

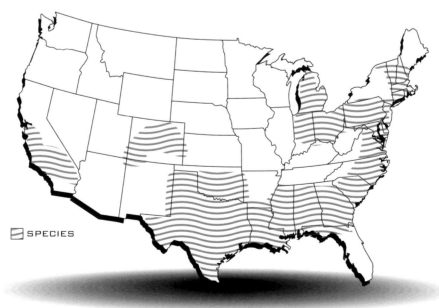

▨ SPECIES

MONTHS OF ALLERGENIC SEVERITY

| JAN | FEB | MAR | APR | MAY | JNE | JLY | AUG | SEPT | OCT | NOV | DEC |

◣ BOTANICAL NAME: *Pennisetum setaceum*
COMMON NAME: FOUNTAIN GRASS
USDA ZONES: 1, 2, 3, 4, 5, 6, 7, 8, 9, 10

DEGREE OF ALLERGENIC SEVERITY: Occasional

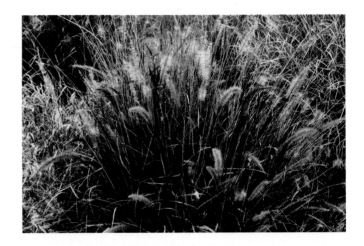

AREAS OF KNOWN PLANT

EXISTENCE:
Fountain grass is an introduced plant that is considered "locally common" within its USDA zones. Fountain grass has escaped cultivation and has naturalized in sandy places of California and possibly other states. Not much information on this plant exists outside of cultivation. This could be a problem plant in the future. Fountain grass is used as an annual in colder regions.

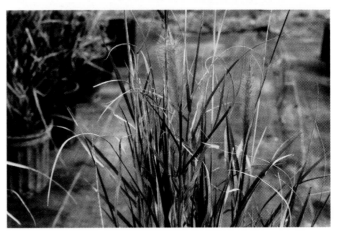

NATURAL CONCENTRATIONS:
Fountain grass has been found growing outside of cultivation in scattered areas of San Diego to Ventura County in California. It is also reported in Alameda County in California. Other species of *Pennisetum* have mildly escaped cultivation in Michigan and Texas.

AREAS OF KNOWN ALLERGY

RELIEF:
Unpopulated natural areas in the Northwest.

PARTIAL RELIEF:
Relief and or partial relief can probably be found in most unpopulated areas not supporting a Mediterranean climate. I suspect we will see a lot more of this plant escaping cultivation and establishing itself in rural and unpopulated areas.

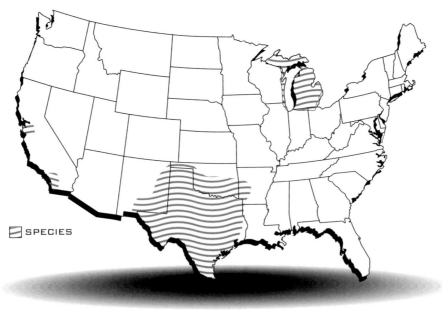

▨ SPECIES

MONTHS OF ALLERGENIC SEVERITY

| JAN | FEB | MAR | APR | MAY | JNE | JLY | AUG | SEPT | OCT | NOV | DEC |

BOTANICAL NAME: *Phalaris arundinacea*
COMMON NAME: **CANARY GRASS**
USDA ZONES: 1, 2, 3, 4, 5, 6, 7, 8

DEGREE OF ALLERGENIC SEVERITY: Occasional

AREAS OF KNOWN PLANT

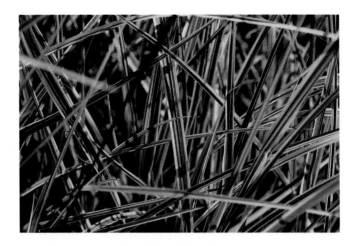

EXISTENCE:
Canary grass can be found growing on wet slopes, moist areas, below 5,000 feet in elevation. In the East, canary grass is found along shores, swales and meadows. It is also mildly used as an ornamental shrub. It may be mildly "locally common."

NATURAL CONCENTRATIONS:
Canary grass grows from Alaska south to east Maryland, North Carolina, Kentucky, Illinois, Missouri, Oklahoma, Arizona, New Mexico and California, (San Joaquin Valley).

AREAS OF KNOWN ALLERGY

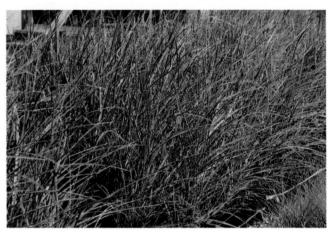

RELIEF:
Above 5,000 feet in elevation.

PARTIAL RELIEF:
Texas to Florida, coastal California, southwestern Arizona.

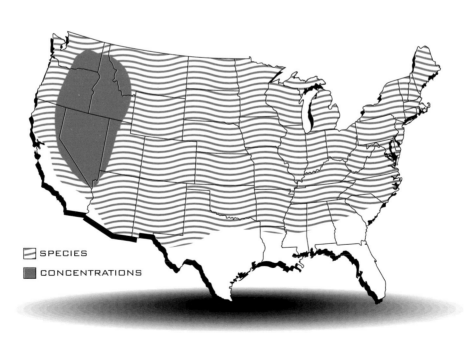

SPECIES
CONCENTRATIONS

MONTHS OF ALLERGENIC SEVERITY

JAN	FEB	MAR	APR	MAY	JNE	JLY	AUG	SEPT	OCT	NOV	DEC

BOTANICAL NAME: *Sambucus spp.*
COMMON NAME: **RED, BLUE,**
AMERICAN ELDERBERRY
USDA ZONES: 4, 5, 6, 7, 8, 9

DEGREE OF ALLERGENIC SEVERITY: Occasional

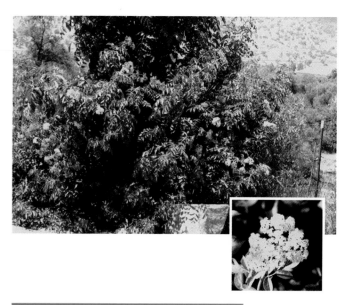

AREAS OF KNOWN PLANT

EXISTENCE:
Elderberries are native to California, Eastern United States and northward into Canada. Elderberries are cultivated and used in the urban and rural landscapes. Consider them mildly "locally common." Naturally, elderberries grow in damp, rich soils in woodlands and openings, roadsides, waste places, and at times in rocky soil.

NATURAL CONCENTRATIONS:
Elderberries grow in catered bunches throughout the Sierra Nevada Mountains and foothills and along the Coast Range Mountains in California. Elderberries also extend into western Washington, Oregon and Canada. Elderberries has been spotted growing in limited parts of Idaho, Nevada, Utah, Arizona, New Mexico, Colorado, Wyoming and Montana.

In the East, elderberries grow from Nova Scotia to New England, south to Virginia, Georgia, Louisiana, Oklahoma, Florida, and Texas.

AREAS OF KNOWN ALLERGY

RELIEF:
Dry desert areas of the West, south Florida Keys, southern Oklahoma to northern Alabama and central Tennessee, north Texas, lower Rio Grande Valley, south interior plains, and the hill country of central Texas

PARTIAL RELIEF:
Most Western states east of California, Washington, and Oregon that are dry and unpopulated.

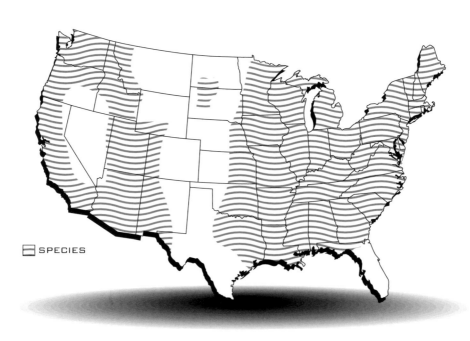

SPECIES

MONTHS OF ALLERGENIC SEVERITY

| JAN | FEB | MAR | APR | MAY | JNE | JLY | AUG | SEPT | OCT | NOV | DEC |

BOTANICAL NAME: *Syringa spp.*
COMMON NAME: **LILACS**
USDA ZONES: 2, 3, 4, 5, 6, 7, 8

DEGREE OF ALLERGENIC SEVERITY: Moderate

AREAS OF KNOWN PLANT

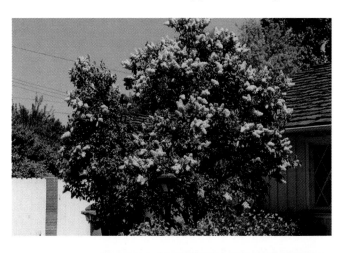

EXISTENCE:
Lilacs are not native to the United States and have not naturalized to any extent. Therefore, consider lilacs "locally common" in their USDA plant zones. Lilacs need a good winter chill to bloom properly and profusely.

CONCENTRATIONS:
Lilacs can be found mostly in gardens and landscapes in the middle to northern latitudes throughout the United States. Many old-time gardens will have lilacs in them.

AREAS OF KNOWN ALLERGY

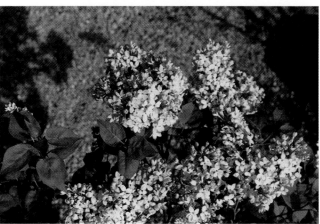

RELIEF:
Areas of no winter chill. Southern Oregon coast to San Diego. Most desert areas of California, Arizona, New Mexico, and Texas. Through the lower half of the Gulf States along the Atlantic coast to southern Virginia.

PARTIAL RELIEF:
Central areas of Arizona, New Mexico, Texas, the Gulf States, Georgia, South Carolina, and North Carolina.

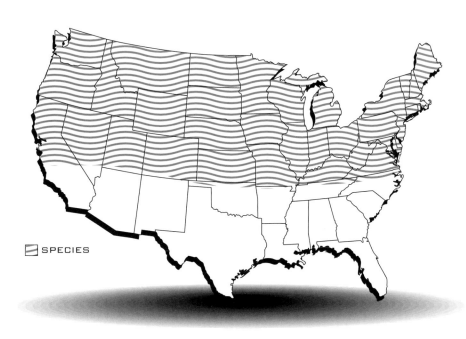

SPECIES

MONTHS OF ALLERGENIC SEVERITY

| JAN | FEB | MAR | APR | MAY | JNE | JLY | AUG | SEPT | OCT | NOV | DEC |

BOTANICAL NAME: *Acacia spp.*
COMMON NAME: ACACIAS
USDA ZONES: 8, 9

DEGREE OF ALLERGENIC SEVERITY: Moderate

AREAS OF KNOWN PLANT

EXISTENCE:
There are many varieties of acacias mostly from Australia. A few are native to the United States, mostly in the West. Naturally, acacias generally grow in desert or desert grassland areas in washes, slopes, dry mesas, plains, low, and rocky canyons and rocky woods in mostly limestone or poor soils. Acacias usually grow in mass numbers causing dense thickets. They are a very popular landscape plant and have been for many years. They can be seen growing in cities, towns and farms in almost all areas within their USDA zones. So consider them "locally common."

NATURAL CONCENTRATIONS:
Acacia trees grow naturally in the warmer desert areas of the southeastern Mojave Desert of California extending northward into Clark County in Nevada and near St. George in the southwest corner of Utah. In Arizona the acacias mainly grow in the lower half of the state primarily in the Mojave, Colorado and Arizona Deserts. Acacias can also be seen in the Chihuahuan Desert and surrounding areas near Albuquerque in New Mexico, Arkansas, to south Kansas, southwest Missouri and on down into the central, southwest and Trans-Pecos area in Texas. Their elevation extends to 5,000 feet.

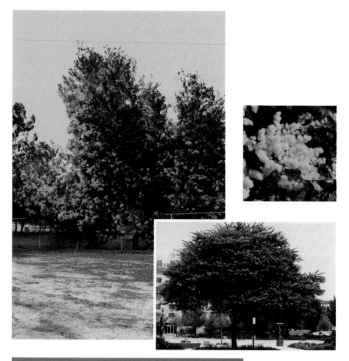

AREAS OF KNOWN ALLERGY

RELIEF:
In USDA zones 1, 2, 3, 4, 5 or higher elevations generally above 5,000 feet, and Sierra Nevada Mountains in California, Idaho, eastern Washington and Oregon, northern Nevada, Montana, Wyoming, Colorado, northern Texas, all states north (inland) of the Gulf States and southeastern states near Georgetown in South Carolina.

PARTIAL RELIEF:
Most of Utah and northern Arizona, northern areas of New Mexico, Louisiana, and Florida.

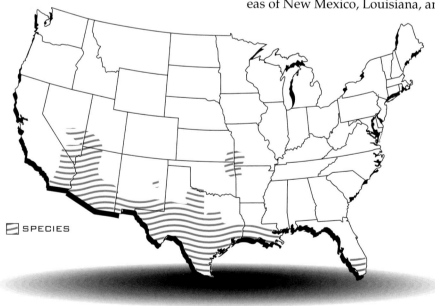

☐ SPECIES

MONTHS OF ALLERGENIC SEVERITY

| JAN | FEB | MAR | APR | MAY | JNE | JLY | AUG | SEPT | OCT | NOV | DEC |

BOTANICAL NAME: *Acer spp.*
COMMON NAME: **MAPLES**
USDA ZONES: 3, 4, 5, 6, 7, 8, 9

DEGREE OF ALLERGENIC SEVERITY: Occasional to moderate depending on the species. Box elder (*Acer negundo*) is thought to be one of the worst of the maples.

AREAS OF KNOWN PLANT

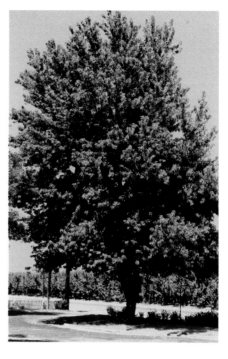
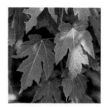
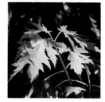

EXISTENCE:
There are many native species of maple trees which can be found in areas of moist soil of valley and upland slopes, near streams, flood plains, swamps and riverbanks, and as an understory plant in mixed hardwood forests. Native and introduced maples have escaped nonnative areas especially along the east and southern coast, in waste places and along roadsides. Maples are very abundant, so consider them "locally common" throughout the populated areas within their climate zones. In the urban landscape, maples are used as street trees, in parks, schools and about the urban landscape.

NATURAL CONCENTRATIONS:
Native or naturalized maple trees can be found growing in the Rocky Mountains, from New Mexico north into Canada, southern Arizona, Wasscach Mountains of Utah, eastern Texas, Pacific Northwest, northern California and Lake Tahoe area, Elko and Lincoln Counties and in the Quinn Mountains of Nevada. Maple trees can also be found growing in the Panamint, Inyo-White Mountains, on the eastern slope of the Sierra Nevada Mountains, Santa Barbara and Kern Counties of California, and north of California to Alaska. Maples generally grow naturally at elevations between 4,000 and 8,000 feet.

In the East, maples grow throughout most of the states, including the Adirondack Virgin Forest in New York, Appalachian Mountains, Iowa, and Florida.

AREAS OF KNOWN ALLERGY

RELIEF:
Great Basin in Nevada.

PARTIAL RELIEF:
Elevations above 8,000 feet or below 4,000 feet in unpopulated areas. Also, unpopulated areas of northwestern Texas, Utah, southeastern New Mexico, and northern Arizona.

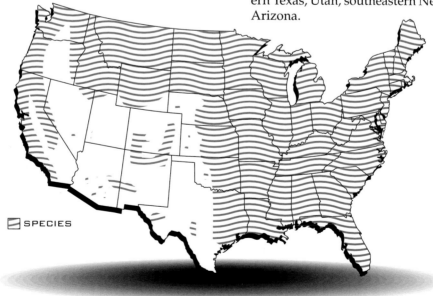

SPECIES

MONTHS OF ALLERGENIC SEVERITY

| JAN | FEB | MAR | APR | MAY | JNE | JLY | AUG | SEPT | OCT | NOV | DEC |

BOTANICAL NAME: *Aesculus spp.*
COMMON NAME: BUCKEYE, HORSECHESTNUT
USDA ZONES: 5, 6, 7, 8, 9

DEGREE OF ALLERGENIC SEVERITY: Moderate

AREAS OF KNOWN PLAN

EXISTENCE:
In the West, buckeye trees grow on moist or dry hillsides and canyons in foothill or chaparral communities, often in association with oak trees. In the East, buckeye trees grow in woods and thickets or stream banks, coastal plains, bottom lands or lower mountains. They are used infrequently as an ornamental but are only slightly considered "locally common." Buckeye trees can loose their leaves in the summer months (summer deciduous).

NATURAL CONCENTRATIONS:
Naturally buckeyes are found in the Sierra Nevada and Coast Range Mountains to 4,000 feet in elevation in California. This tree is not found naturally in any other western state, except for eastern Texas.
In the East, buckeye trees grow from Pennsylvania, Ohio, Michigan south to Iowa and Nebraska, south into Alabama, Mississippi, Arkansas, Oklahoma, Florida to Louisiana, north into Georgia, Virginia, West Virginia, and Kentucky.

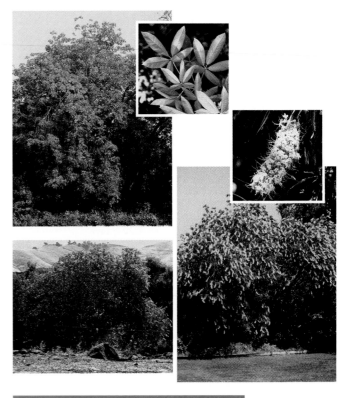

AREAS OF KNOWN ALLERGY

RELIEF:
USDA zones 1, 2, 3, 4. Natural areas in all western states except California. Elevations above 4,500 feet.

PARTIAL RELIEF:
Northwest, southern California, most areas in the San Joaquin Valley, southern Florida, West Texas and New England states.

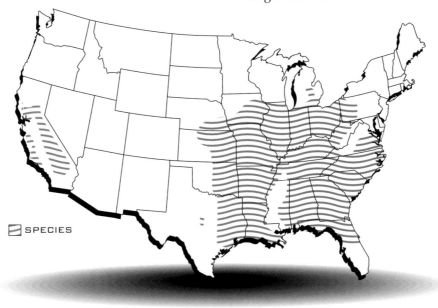

SPECIES

MONTHS OF ALLERGENIC SEVERITY

| JAN | FEB | MAR | APR | MAY | JNE | JLY | AUG | SEPT | OCT | NOV | DEC |

BOTANICAL NAME: *Ailanthus altissima*
COMMON NAME: **TREE-OF-HEAVEN**
USDA ZONES: 5, 6, 7, 8

DEGREE OF ALLERGENIC SEVERITY: Occasional to moderate

AREAS OF KNOWN PLANT

EXISTENCE:
The tree-of-heaven is an introduced tree from China during the gold rush era in California; it established itself along rivers and streams, city lots, ditches, and waste places. This tree is very fast growing, spreads easily, and has an objectionable odor. It has been used in the past as a street tree, for wind breaks, shade, and in areas where other trees will not grow. Tree-of-heaven will be a problem tree in the near future.

NATURAL CONCENTRATIONS:
The tree-of-heaven has spread from California to the southern Rocky Mountains and Oregon. In California it has established itself in the mountain areas and San Joaquin and Sacramento Valleys and over to the coastal areas. In the Southwest it has escaped along waterways and areas of sustainable moisture and is reported to be established and spreading in southern New Mexico.
In the East, this tree has escaped cultivation in Massachusetts, Iowa, and north to south Ontario in Canada.

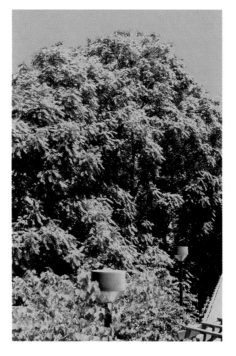

AREAS OF KNOWN ALLERGY

RELIEF:
Little information is available on the spread of this tree. It is aggressive and will tolerate many harsh conditions so expect this tree to keep on spreading.

PARTIAL RELIEF:
USDA zones 1, 2, 3. Natural, unpopulated areas of little or no water, i.e., the Great Basin, and other desert areas.

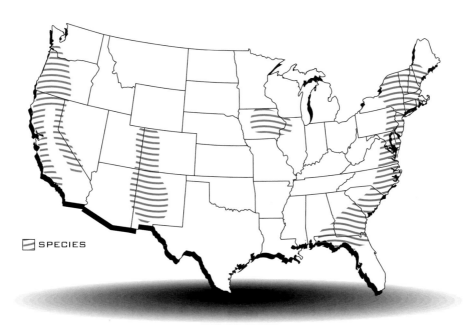

SPECIES

MONTHS OF ALLERGENIC SEVERITY

| JAN | FEB | MAR | APR | MAY | JNE | JLY | AUG | SEPT | OCT | NOV | DEC |

■ BOTANICAL NAME: *Alnus spp.*
COMMON NAME: **WHITE ALDER,**
THINLEAF ALDER,
USDA ZONES: 2, 3, 4, 5, 6, 7, 8, 9

DEGREE OF ALLERGENIC SEVERITY: Moderate.

AREAS OF KNOWN PLANT

EXISTENCE:
Both the native and introduced varieties of alders have found their way into the United States home landscapes and are considered "locally common" throughout. Naturally, alders can be found along stream beds, lakes, and marshy meadows in the many mountainous regions of the United States.

NATURAL CONCENTRATIONS:
Native alders can be found throughout the Sierra Nevada Mountains in California, the Cascade and other mountainous areas of Oregon, the Rocky Mountains in Colorado, extending northward into Alaska. Alders are also found naturally in Utah's Wasatch Mountain Range and Raft River Mountains, and western Colorado. Alders also grow on both sides of the Grand Canyon, and mountainous areas of southeast Arizona, south and western New Mexico and northeast Nevada. In the East, alders grow almost everywhere including the higher mountains of New England, northern New York, and west Connecticut, south Delaware, east shore of Maryland near sea level, parts of Indiana and Illinois, Michigan, Wisconsin, Minnesota, West Virginia to northeast Iowa and northeast North Dakota, Missouri, Arkansas, Oklahoma (at 700 feet elevation), southern states to north Florida, west to east

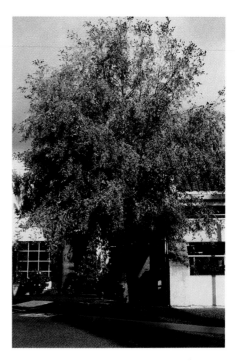

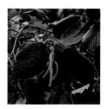

Texas, and north to southeast Kansas, and most of Canada.

AREAS OF KNOWN ALLERGY

RELIEF:
Natural, unpopulated, and low elevations in hot dry areas throughout the United States.

PARTIAL RELIEF:
Desert climates, unpopulated, eastern side of Montana, western Colorado and Wyoming, and east New Mexico, southern Florida, western parts of the Midwest.

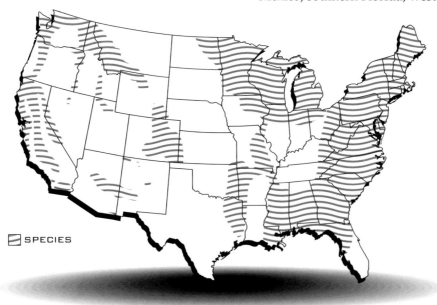

▱ SPECIES

MONTHS OF ALLERGENIC SEVERITY

| JAN | FEB | MAR | APR | MAY | JNE | JLY | AUG | SEPT | OCT | NOV | DEC |

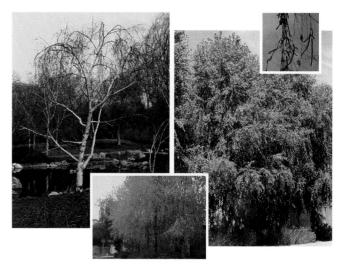

BOTANICAL NAME: *Betula spp.*
COMMON NAME: **WHITE BIRCH,**
WATER BIRCH
USDA ZONES: 2, 3, 4, 5, 6, 7, 8, 9

DEGREE OF ALLERGENIC SEVERITY: Moderate to high

AREAS OF KNOWN PLANT

EXISTENCE:

Both native and introduced varieties of birch trees are extremely widespread in United States landscape. They are considered "locally common" throughout the populated areas in their respective USDA climate zones. Fortunately, birch trees have a very short pollination period, approximately one week. Naturally, birch trees are found along streams, rivers, and wet areas with an occasional growth in drier areas. They are associated with poplars, alders, willows, aspen, pine, maples, red oaks or in pure stands.

NATURAL CONCENTRATIONS:

Birch trees can be found in almost every city in the United States that will support its climatic needs. Naturally occurring birch trees can be found in eastern Washington and Oregon. Also, found in Utah growing along streams that flow into the desert and in the higher mountain ranges (5,000 to 8,000 feet elevation). In California birch trees are found in the Sierra Nevada Mountains, White, Panamint and Warner Mountains, Tulare, Modoc, Siskyou and Humbolt counties. Other areas include northern New Mexico, northern Idaho, western Montana, south and western Wyoming, central Colorado and spotty in eastern Nevada.

In the East, birch trees grow heavily from Maine south to northern Florida, extending west to east Texas, eastern Oklahoma, Missouri, eastern and northern Iowa, and Minnesota eastward through the Great Lakes. One species of birch (Betula uber) is reported to grow only in southwest Virginia in Smyth County at 2,750 feet in elevation.

AREAS OF KNOWN ALLERGY

RELIEF:

Unpopulated, natural drier areas of southern Arizona, New Mexico, central and western Texas and the central Midwest, southern Florida and Louisiana.

PARTIAL RELIEF:

Unpopulated, natural dry areas of southern California, western Washington and Oregon, eastern Montana, Wyoming, and below 3,000 feet in elevation.

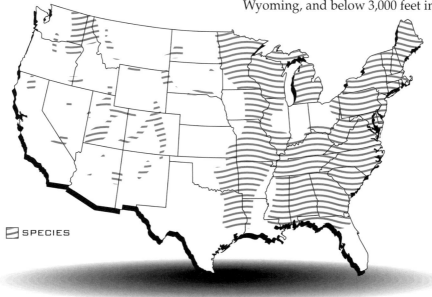

☐ SPECIES

MONTHS OF ALLERGENIC SEVERITY

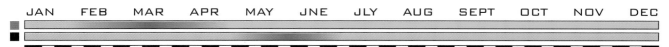

JAN	FEB	MAR	APR	MAY	JNE	JLY	AUG	SEPT	OCT	NOV	DEC

■ WESTERN STATES ■ EASTERN STATES

BOTANICAL NAME: *Calocedrus (Libocedrus) decurrens*
COMMON NAME: **INCENSE CEDAR**
USDA ZONES: 5, 6, 7, 8

DEGREE OF ALLERGENIC SEVERITY: Moderate

AREAS OF KNOWN PLANT

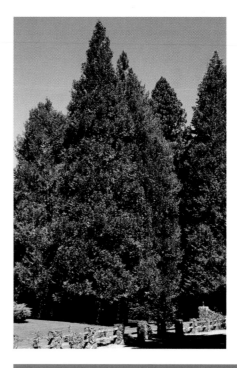

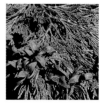

EXISTENCE:

Naturally, the incense cedar grows in moist western slope mountain soils, in mixed evergreen forests at elevations between 2,400 and 8,200 feet. The popularity in the aromatic fragrance of the wood has led to the use of this tree outside its natural environment, so consider this tree to be mildly "locally common" in many communities within its USDA climate zones.

NATURAL CONCENTRATIONS:

The incense cedar is mostly found in the Sierra Nevada Mountains (Yosemite Valley and eastern slope near Reno, Nevada) and in the northern Warner Mountains of California. It grows sparingly in southern California. In Oregon the incense cedar is found on the southeast slope of Mt. Hood and in the southern Cascade Mountains. People who are allergic to incense cedar trees and travel into these regions will often experience headaches. Incense cedar seldom grows in pure stands.

In the East, incense cedar is planted ornamentally in the New England and Mid-Atlantic states. It is not native in the East.

AREAS OF KNOWN ALLERGY

RELIEF:

Unpopulated or natural areas of Idaho, Montana, Wyoming, Colorado, southern Nevada, Arizona, New Mexico, Utah, and natural areas below 2,400 feet elevation. Natural areas in the Midwest and East.

PARTIAL RELIEF:

Eastern Oregon, coastal Oregon, areas of northern California below 2,400 feet or above 8,200 feet elevation.

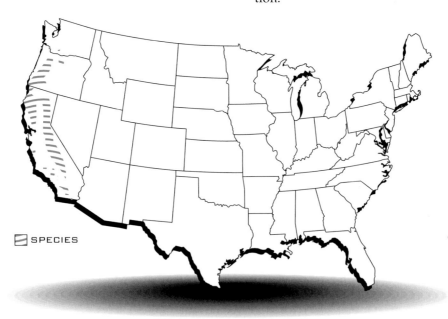

SPECIES

MONTHS OF ALLERGENIC SEVERITY

| JAN | FEB | MAR | APR | MAY | JNE | JLY | AUG | SEPT | OCT | NOV | DEC |

BOTANICAL NAME: *Chamaecyparis lawsoniana*
COMMON NAME: **PORT-ORFORD CEDAR,
LAWSON CYPRESS**
USDA ZONES: 7, 8

DEGREE OF ALLERGENIC SEVERITY: Occasional

AREAS OF KNOWN PLANT

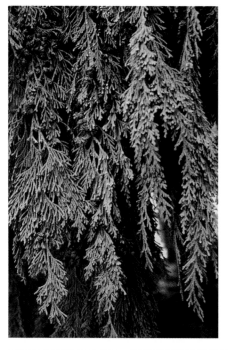

EXISTENCE:
Naturally, port-orford cedar grows in moist slopes, mountains and canyons often on serpentine soil in coastal coniferous forests or mixed evergreen forests.

NATURAL CONCENTRATIONS:
The port-orford cedar grow mostly in western Oregon, extending into Siskiyou, Shasta, to Humboldt and Del Norte Counties in northwestern California. The port-orford cedar grows below 4,800 feet in elevation. Its boundaries are expanding because of its ornamental appeal. Related eastern species grow in cool acid bogs from Maine to Florida and in Mississippi.

AREAS OF KNOWN ALLERGY

RELIEF:
USDA zones 1 to 6. Natural areas in Montana, Wyoming, Utah, Nevada, central and southern California, Arizona, and New Mexico. This species doesn't grow naturally in the Midwest or East coast, however, it is used as an ornamental tree, so suspect it to appear occasionally in cities and towns within its USDA zones.

PARTIAL RELIEF:
Natural areas of Idaho, Western Oregon and Washington, elevations above 5,000 feet.

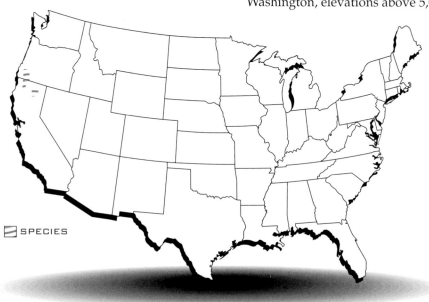

☐ SPECIES

MONTHS OF ALLERGENIC SEVERITY

| JAN | FEB | MAR | APR | MAY | JNE | JLY | AUG | SEPT | OCT | NOV | DEC |

■ BOTANICAL NAME: *Cupressus spp.*
COMMON NAME: **ARIZONA, MONTEREY, SARGENT, PIOTE, MACNAB, MODOC, GOWEN, ITALIAN CYPRESS**
USDA ZONES: 5, 6, 7, 8, 9

DEGREE OF ALLERGENIC SEVERITY: Moderate

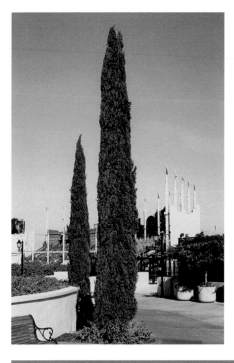
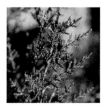

AREAS OF KNOWN PLANT

EXISTENCE:
The many different species of cypress trees have found their way into our western landscapes and they are considered "locally common" in many states, especially California, Arizona, and New Mexico. Naturally, cypress trees like a wide variety of soils and climates. Some grow best only near the coast while others thrive in mountainous regions and high desert areas. They are generally found at elevations below 2,600 feet except for the Arizona Cypress which grows naturally at elevations of 3,200 to 8,700 feet.

NATURAL CONCENTRATIONS:
The different species of natural cypress trees are quite specific in their habitat and occupy a small geographic area. Most of the native cypress trees are found in California, ranging from the northern inland border with Oregon to the Monterey coast and San Diego area. In the Southwest, cypress can be found in scattered parts of central and southeast Arizona, and southwest New Mexico.

AREAS OF KNOWN ALLERGY

RELIEF:
Natural, unpopulated areas of Washington, Idaho, Montana, Wyoming, Colorado, Utah, Nevada, northern Oregon, and New Mexico. Natural non-populated areas of the Midwest and Eastern United States.

PARTIAL RELIEF:
Natural areas of the Sierra Nevada Mountains south of Lake Tahoe, California, northern Arizona, and New Mexico.

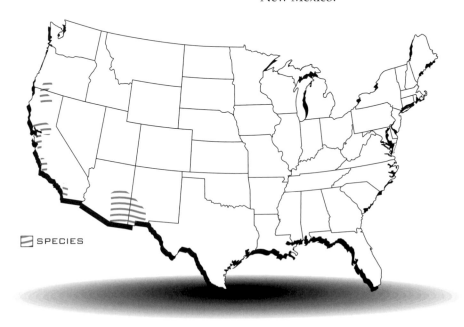

▤ SPECIES

MONTHS OF ALLERGENIC SEVERITY

JAN	FEB	MAR	APR	MAY	JNE	JLY	AUG	SEPT	OCT	NOV	DEC

BOTANICAL NAME: *Fraxinus spp.*
COMMON NAME: ASH
USDA ZONES: 3, 4, 5, 6, 7, 8, 9

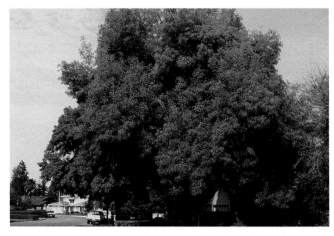

DEGREE OF ALLERGENIC SEVERITY: Occasional to moderate.

AREAS OF KNOWN PLANT

EXISTENCE:
Ash trees grow naturally in mountains along rivers, streams, canyons, rich uplands to lowlands, and areas of moist soil and swamp forests. Occasionally they can be found in desert grasslands where there is an underground water supply or dry rocky bluffs of limestone. They are quite a diverse species of tree. Ash trees grow among red alders, black cottonwoods, willows, and oaks. In populated areas, ash trees are planted throughout, mostly for their quick shade qualities and are considered "locally common." One ash species is a hybrid cross (Raywood ash) and doesn't produce pollen it is considered allergy-free (see chapter 5).

NATURAL CONCENTRATIONS:
Ash trees can be found naturally growing in the Sierra Nevada and Coastal mountain ranges up to 11,000 feet in California. They can also be found growing in western Colorado, lower and eastern Utah, in the Grand Canyon National Park and Coronado National Forest near Nogalez in Arizona, and in the northern New Mexico mountains between 4,500 feet and 7,000 feet. In the Pacific Northwest, ash trees can be found growing west of the Cascade Mountains in Washington and Oregon.
In the East, ash trees grow almost everywhere except southern Florida and the southern tip of Texas.

They also grow in Canada. A few specific areas where ash trees grow include warm valleys in New England, bottomlands or wet shores in Florida to east Texas, Coastal Plain to Virginia, dry or moist rich woods of Canada to Minnesota, Michigan and Wisconsin, Arbuckle Mountains of Oklahoma, Limestone bluff in Texas, Hardwood Limestone forest from Ohio to northwest Georgia, Great Plains, southern Maryland, and southern Appalachians.

AREAS OF KNOWN ALLERGY

RELIEF:
Natural areas of western Montana, western Wyoming Idaho, and southern Florida.

PARTIAL RELIEF:
Natural, unpopulated, dry soil areas of central and northern Nevada, central and eastern Oregon and Washington, Colorado, and southern Florida.

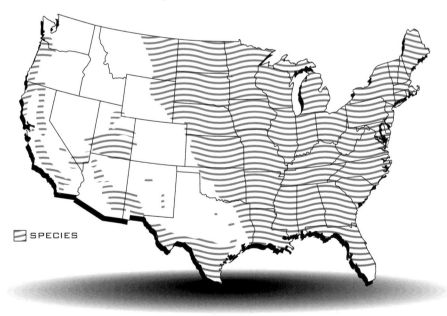

▱ SPECIES

MONTHS OF ALLERGENIC SEVERITY

| JAN | FEB | MAR | APR | MAY | JNE | JLY | AUG | SEPT | OCT | NOV | DEC |

BOTANICAL NAME: *Juglans spp.*
COMMON NAME: **WALNUT**
USDA ZONES: 3, 4, 5, 6, 7, 8, 9

DEGREE OF ALLERGENIC SEVERITY: High to very high

AREAS OF KNOWN PLANT

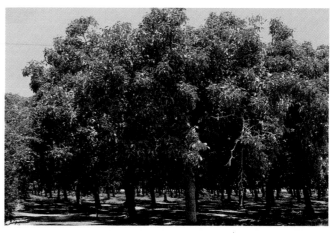

EXISTENCE:

Walnuts are not often used as an ornamental tree. They are widely used as an agricultural crop. It's becoming a practice in California to keep many of the trees when walnut orchards are being converted to subdivision property. The remaining trees are left as established shade trees on the lots. Anyone who suffers from allergies caused by walnuts would no doubt be affected by entering this type of environment. Naturally, walnuts can be found growing in moist or dry gravelly to deep loam soils in canyons, mountains, bottom land and flood plains, grasslands, foothills, deserts and forests, along streams and rivers, between 2,000 and 7,600 feet elevation.

NATURAL CONCENTRATIONS:

Native walnut species can be found growing in the California Coast Range Mountains from the greater San Francisco area southward to Santa Barbara and picking up again in and around the San Diego area. Other concentrations of walnuts can be found along the Sacramento River, especially below the Lake Tahoe area, and agriculturally in the San Joaquin and Sacramento Valleys. It's also found along stream banks in canyons of central and southern New Mexico and Arizona, Oak Creek near Flagstaff in Arizona, on the Colorado plateau.

In the East, walnuts grow from southeastern Canada south to northern Georgia, and northwest Florida west to central Texas, north to southeast South Dakota, eastern Minnesota, southern Michigan, and Canada. Specific areas include northern Michigan peninsula, Appalachian Mountains and adjoining foothills near Fort Worth in Texas.

AREAS OF KNOWN ALLERGY

RELIEF:

Natural, unpopulated areas of Washington, Oregon, Idaho, Montana, Wyoming, Utah, Colorado, eastern Georgia and South Carolina, northern Michigan and Minnesota, southern Florida, the Gulf Coast, southern California coast, lower Rio Grande Valley, high deserts of Arizona, medium to high desert of California and southern Nevada, medium to low deserts in California and Arizona (California to Arizona).

PARTIAL RELIEF:

Generally, walnuts are not found growing above 7,600 feet. Central Georgia, South Carolina, central Nebraska, northern Maine, and New Hampshire.

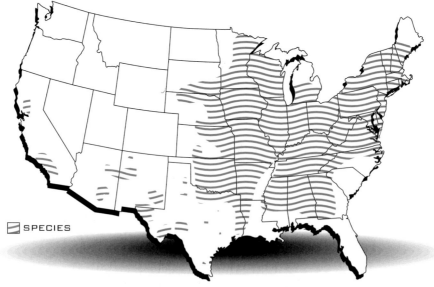

SPECIES

MONTHS OF ALLERGENIC SEVERITY

| JAN | FEB | MAR | APR | MAY | JNE | JLY | AUG | SEPT | OCT | NOV | DEC |

■ WESTERN STATES ■ EASTERN STATES

BOTANICAL NAME: *Liquidambar styraciflua*
COMMON NAME: **SWEET GUM,**
LIQUIDAMBAR
USDA ZONES: 5, 6, 7, 8, 9

DEGREE OF ALLERGENIC SEVERITY: Occasional

AREAS OF KNOWN PLANT

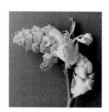

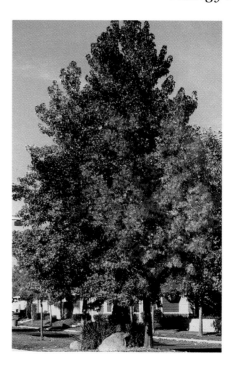

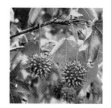

EXISTENCE:
The sweet gum tree is native to the Eastern Un-tied States and is strictly used as an ornamental landscape tree in the West. The sweet gum has not naturalized itself in the western wilderness; however, this tree is quite popular in western cities and towns, so consider it "locally common" within its USDA climate zones.

In the East, sweet gum can be found in swampy woods, rich and moist valleys and lower slope soils usually in mixed woodlands. They are quick to fill in old fields after clear cutting or logging.

NATURAL CONCENTRATIONS:
Naturally sweet gum grows from southeast New York, southwest Connecticut (Fairfield County) and eastern Pennsylvania, south to Cape Canaveral and Tampa Bay in Florida, east Texas, Arkansas and Missouri to southern Illinois, Ohio and Indiana, lower Appalachian Mountains (to 3000'), Mississippi Delta region.

AREAS OF KNOWN ALLERGY

RELIEF:
USDA zones 1, 2, 3, 4. Natural and unpopulated areas in the Western United States, Southern Florida, extreme northern and eastern states, Iowa, Nebraska, central and western Missouri, Oklahoma.

PARTIAL RELIEF:
Natural areas bordering populated areas in the West. In the East, central Florida, central and northern Ohio, Indiana, Illinois, eastern West Virginia and Tennessee, western Maryland, and Pennsylvania.

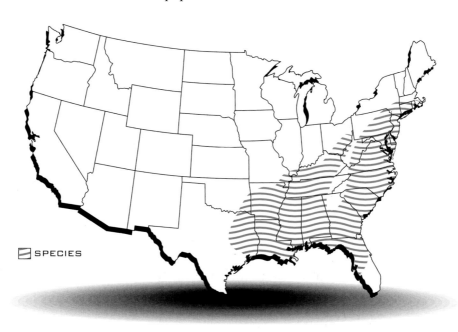

SPECIES

MONTHS OF ALLERGENIC SEVERITY

| JAN | FEB | MAR | APR | MAY | JNE | JLY | AUG | SEPT | OCT | NOV | DEC |

■ WESTERN STATES ■ EASTERN STATES

BOTANICAL NAME: *Morus spp.*
COMMON NAME: **RED MULBERRY,**
TEXAS MULBERRY
USDA ZONES: 5, 6, 7, 8, 9, 10

DEGREE OF ALLERGENIC SEVERITY: High

AREAS OF KNOWN PLANT

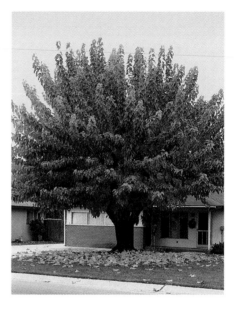
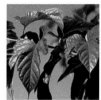

EXISTENCE:
Mulberry trees have been a popular landscape tree for many years; because of this, and their wide range of adaptability, they can be found growing throughout most of the United States, so consider mulberries "locally common" within their USDA zones. Naturally, mulberry trees like moist (generally limestone) soils along streams, rivers, and other water courses, in foothills, wooded mountains, and upper desert areas.

NATURAL CONCENTRATIONS:
The Texas mulberry (*Morus microphylla*) is the only native mulberry tree found in the West. It grows in the valley of Colorado River, into Mexico, and in the mountainous regions of west Texas and south New Mexico, reaching to the Santa Rita Mountains and canyons of the Colorado Plateau in Arizona. The red mulberry (*Morus rubra*) grow sparsely throughout the eastern Midwest to the East coast, from east Texas to east Minnesota, east to New York, south to southern Florida and west to Texas, including the foothills of southern Appalachian Mountains to 2,000 feet, lower Ohio River basin, the shores of Bay Biscayne and Cape Romano in Florida, and Long Island in New York. Its greatest concentrations are in the lower Ohio and Mississippi river basins.

AREAS OF KNOWN ALLERGY

RELIEF:
USDA zones 1, 2, 3. Wyoming, eastern Montana, most of Nevada, Colorado, Idaho, eastern Washington, and Oregon. In the East, relief is noted in interior mountains of Pennsylvania, New York, and St. Lawrence Valley in Canada, upper Michigan, mountains of New England, northern Minnesota, and northwestern Wisconsin.

PARTIAL RELIEF:
Remote unpopulated areas of Washington, Oregon, Idaho, Montana, Wyoming, Colorado, Nevada, Utah, and California. In the East, partial relief may be found in Maine, south Florida and the Keys.

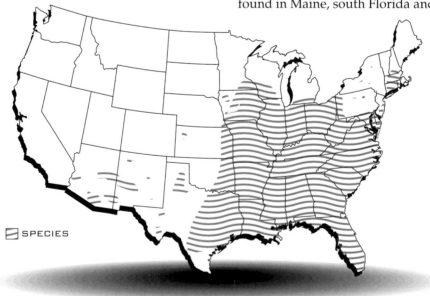

⊟ SPECIES

MONTHS OF ALLERGENIC SEVERITY

| JAN | FEB | MAR | APR | MAY | JNE | JLY | AUG | SEPT | OCT | NOV | DEC |

■ WESTERN STATES ■ EASTERN STATES

BOTANICAL NAME: *Olea europaea*
COMMON NAME: **OLIVE**
USDA ZONES: 8, 9

DEGREE OF ALLERGENIC SEVERITY: High

AREAS OF KNOWN PLANT

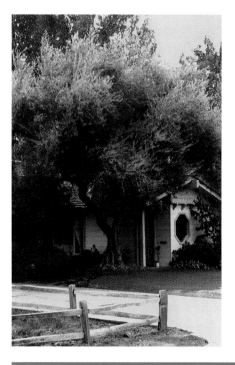

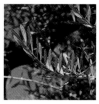

EXISTENCE:
Olive trees were imported to the West and used by the missionaries for oil and fruit. In current times olives are found growing in the western landscapes throughout their USDA climate zones. Olives are also grown as an agricultural commodity. In these areas allergies are higher.

CONCENTRATIONS:
Olives can be found in concentration growing in the San Joaquin Valley in California where they are grown for their oil and fruit. They are also found in populated areas throughout California and Arizona, in milder climates. Olives were grown in Arizona for oil and fruit some years ago but most of the old groves have been removed or the remaining trees have been incorporated into the city landscapes, especially in and around Phoenix and Scottsdale.

Olives trees are not found in the eastern United States.

AREAS OF KNOWN ALLERGY

RELIEF:
Cold climate areas. USDA zones 1 to 7. Oregon, Washington, Utah, Wyoming, Colorado, Montana, Idaho, Nevada, Midwest, and Eastern states.

PARTIAL RELIEF:
Outlying areas of USDA zone 7.

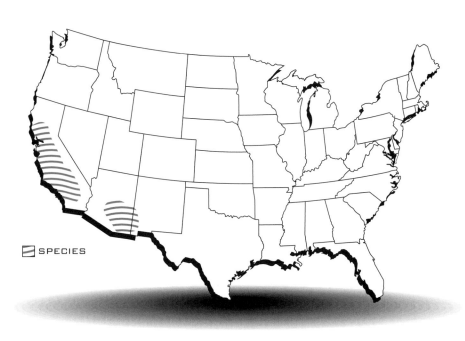

SPECIES

MONTHS OF ALLERGENIC SEVERITY

| JAN | FEB | MAR | APR | MAY | JNE | JLY | AUG | SEPT | OCT | NOV | DEC |

BOTANICAL NAME: *Platanus spp.*
COMMON NAME: **SYCAMORE**
USDA ZONES: 5, 6, 7, 8, 9

DEGREE OF ALLERGENIC SEVERITY: High

AREAS OF KNOWN PLANT

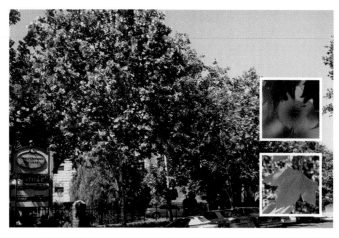

EXISTENCE:

Sycamore trees are scattered across the United States in cities and towns and should be considered "locally common" almost everywhere. Naturally, sycamore trees like moist to wet soils and grow mostly along rivers, streams, and lakes, from the mountains and foothills to fertile valley floors and desert grasslands. Sycamore trees often grow with oaks, cottonwoods, and willows.

NATURAL CONCENTRATIONS:

The California sycamore (*Platanus racemosa*) tree is concentrated naturally in lower elevations in the Sierra Nevada Mountains and along the California coastal range extending into the valley floors predominantly along the water courses that flow out of the mountains. The California sycamore extends into Baja California in Mexico. The Arizona sycamore (*Platanus wrightii*) grows mostly in the mountainous, wet areas of central and northern Arizona 2,000 feet to 6,000 feet including Sycamore Canyon near Williams, and Oak Creek Canyon near Flagstaff, extending to the southeastern border, spilling into canyons of southwestern New Mexico, western Texas, and southward into Mexico, often in association with oaks.

In the East, sycamore trees (*Platanus occidentalis*) grow throughout most of the states from southeastern Maine, to northern Vermont into Canada, and south through Michigan to central and southern Iowa, bordering the eastern parts of Nebraska, Kansas, Oklahoma and Texas, extending east to central Florida. Concentrations of sycamores are found near the streams of the lower Ohio and Mississippi river basins, coastal areas of the Carolinas, Appalachian Mountains to 2,500 feet.

AREAS OF KNOWN ALLERGY

RELIEF:

USDA zones 1, 2, 3, 4. Natural, unpopulated areas of Nevada, Montana, Wyoming, Colorado, Idaho, North and South Dakota. Easterly, south Florida and the Keys, the lower Rio Grande Valley, Texas, mountains of New England, Minnesota, northern Wisconsin.

PARTIAL RELIEF:

Natural, unpopulated areas of Washington, Oregon, Utah, Central and eastern New Mexico, western Nebraska, Kansas, and Oklahoma.

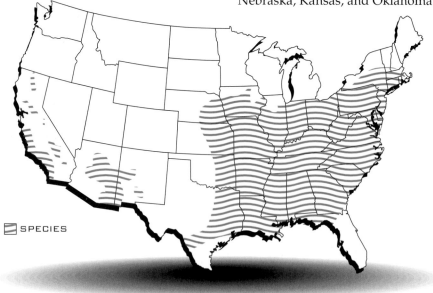

☐ SPECIES

MONTHS OF ALLERGENIC SEVERITY

JAN	FEB	MAR	APR	MAY	JNE	JLY	AUG	SEPT	OCT	NOV	DEC

■ WESTERN STATES ■ EASTERN STATES

BOTANICAL NAME: *Populus spp.*
COMMON NAME: **COTTONWOOD, ASPEN, POPLAR**
USDA ZONES: 2, 3, 4, 5, 6, 7, 8, 9

DEGREE OF ALLERGENIC SEVERITY: Moderate

AREAS OF KNOWN PLANT

EXISTENCE:

Naturally these trees like moist soils and can be found growing along streams, rivers, lakes, and flood plains, often in association with alders, sycamores, willows and oaks, in desert grasslands and into the coniferous forest at most elevations. Cottonwoods, aspen, and poplar are mostly native trees and can be found growing in a wide variety of climates and elevations throughout the United States. These trees are all "locally common" and can be found in almost any city in the United States. They are one of the most planted trees in the desert.

NATURAL CONCENTRATIONS:

Cottonwoods, aspens, and poplars grow in many different climatic conditions, however, the main key to their location is a constant abundance of water, i.e., streams, rivers, lakes, etc. Elevation has little bearing on where they grow. Expect to find one or more of these tree species throughout the West (except in the driest of areas), especially in mountainous areas of Colorado, Utah, Wyoming, Idaho, Washington, Oregon, western slope of the Sierra Nevada mountains, San Diego County in California, and Arizona including the San Francisco Mountains. In Nevada poplar trees are mostly confined to the Reno/Sparks area and along the eastern border. New

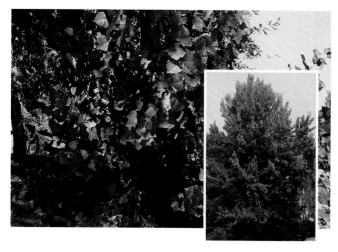

Mexico's cottonwoods, aspens, and poplars are restricted to the wetter mountainous regions.

In the East, poplars are even more widespread except in northeast to southern Florida and parts of the Gulf Coast. Specific areas include mountains of Pennsylvania, Yukon River Valley, Long Island in New York, Piedmont region of Virginia and North Carolina, Apalachicola River valley in Florida, Turtle Mountains in North Dakota, and Black Hills in South Dakota.

AREAS OF KNOWN ALLERGY

RELIEF:

Central and southern Florida.

PARTIAL RELIEF:

Southeastern Oregon down into central Nevada and the desert areas of southern California, lower and dry elevations of New Mexico, eastern Tennessee, and southern Louisiana and Texas.

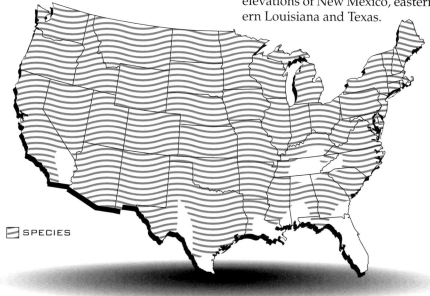

☐ SPECIES

MONTHS OF ALLERGENIC SEVERITY

| JAN | FEB | MAR | APR | MAY | JNE | JLY | AUG | SEPT | OCT | NOV | DEC |

■ WESTERN STATES ■ EASTERN STATES

Allergy Producing Trees

BOTANICAL NAME: *Prosopis spp.*
COMMON NAME: **MESQUITE**
USDA ZONES: 6, 7, 8, 9

DEGREE OF ALLERGENIC SEVERITY: High

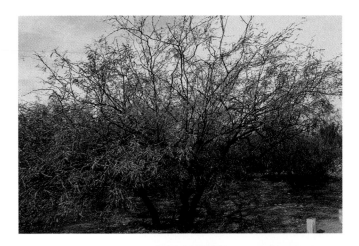

AREAS OF KNOWN PLANT

EXISTENCE:

Mesquite has adapted well in soils of little moisture. Mesquite is slowly being used as an ornamental shrub/tree and can be considered moderately "locally common" in the Southwest and beyond. Naturally, mesquite grows in sandy plains, hills, washes, streams and valleys, usually in large numbers to 5,500 feet in elevation. Mesquite can grow in association with oak trees in some areas. Mesquite is one of the major contributors of allergies in the Southwest.

NATURAL CONCENTRATIONS:

Mesquite grows mostly in desert conditions in southeastern California extending into central Arizona on down into southwestern New Mexico and most of Texas. Mesquite also grows in southern Nevada and Utah. It is reported to be naturalizing in southeast Colorado, Kansas, Louisiana, and possibly Oklahoma. Mesquite is also naturalizing in some areas within its USDA zones.

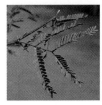
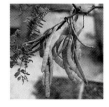

AREAS OF KNOWN ALLERGY

RELIEF:

Washington, Oregon, Montana, Idaho, Wyoming, northern Colorado, states north and east of Kansas, east of Louisiana.

PARTIAL RELIEF:

Central and upper Utah and Nevada, northern California.

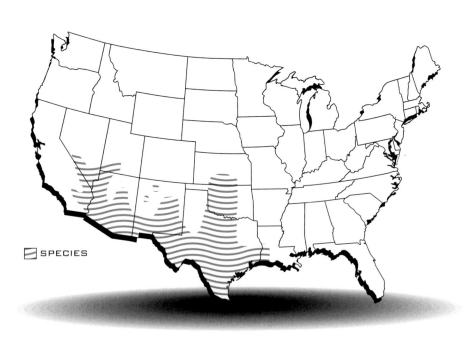

SPECIES

MONTHS OF ALLERGENIC SEVERITY

| JAN | FEB | MAR | APR | MAY | JNE | JLY | AUG | SEPT | OCT | NOV | DEC |

BOTANICAL NAME: *Prunus dulcis*
COMMON NAME: **ALMOND**
USDA ZONES: 6, 7

DEGREE OF ALLERGENIC SEVERITY: High

AREAS OF KNOWN PLANT

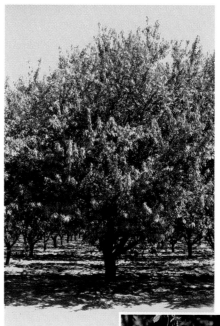

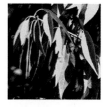

EXISTENCE:
Almonds are mostly grown in the Western United States as an agricultural crop. However, many people grow almonds for nuts in their backyard. They are not considered native and have not escaped cultivation in any appreciable amount.

CONCENTRATIONS:
Almonds can be found in fertile farm grounds in the San Joaquin and Sacramento Valleys in California. They are less known in Arizona and New Mexico and have been noticed in Texas, spreading northeast to Kentucky. Almonds are more of an allergy problem in the West.

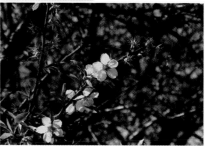

AREAS OF KNOWN ALLERGY

RELIEF:
Humid summer areas and extremely cold areas. This includes Florida and the Gulf Coast and up the eastern seaboard.

PARTIAL RELIEF:
Higher elevations above 6,000 feet.

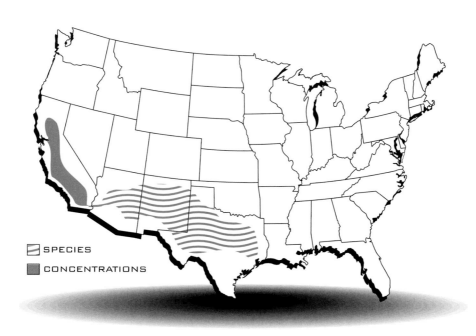

SPECIES

CONCENTRATIONS

MONTHS OF ALLERGENIC SEVERITY

JAN	FEB	MAR	APR	MAY	JNE	JLY	AUG	SEPT	OCT	NOV	DEC

Allergy Producing Trees

■ BOTANICAL NAME: *Quercus spp.*
COMMON NAME: OAK
USDA ZONES: 3, 4, 5, 6, 7, 8, 9

DEGREE OF ALLERGENIC SEVERITY: Occasional to moderate depending on the species

AREAS OF KNOWN PLANT

EXISTENCE:

Oak trees in one species or another can be found throughout most of the United States. They grow in a wide variety of soils, moisture levels, elevations, and climates. There are at least 54 different species of oaks in the United States.

NATURAL CONCENTRATIONS:

California appears to have a wide variety of oak trees growing almost everywhere within the state, extending northward through the western inland portions of Oregon (Mackenzie River) and Washington, including the Columbia River Gorge and in Yakima County. Oaks are also found in Arizona, mountainous portions of Utah and western Colorado, northern and southern New Mexico.

In the East, oaks range throughout. A few specific areas include southern Appalachian Mountains to 4,000 feet, north of the Potomac and Ohio Rivers, near Portage Lake in Michigan, Mississippi Valley, Texas plateau, Stone and Little Stone Mountain in Georgia, near Zuni in Virginia, North Carolina mountains, central Florida, and along Gulf States to the valley of the Neches River in Texas.

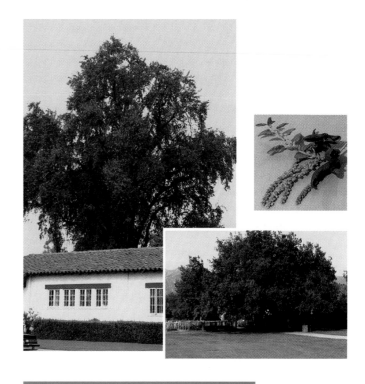

AREAS OF KNOWN ALLERGY

RELIEF:

Natural, unpopulated areas of Idaho, Montana, Great Basin area, central, north and western Wyoming.

PARTIAL RELIEF:

Dry desert areas of New Mexico and Arizona, Montana, Wyoming, possibly South Dakota.

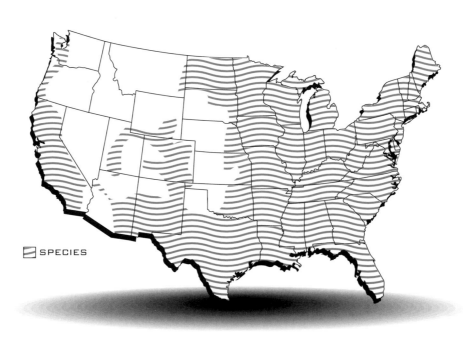

▱ SPECIES

MONTHS OF ALLERGENIC SEVERITY

| JAN | FEB | MAR | APR | MAY | JNE | JLY | AUG | SEPT | OCT | NOV | DEC |

BOTANICAL NAME: *Rhamnus spp.*
COMMON NAME: **BUCKTHORN, COFFEEBERRY**
USDA ZONES: 2, 3, 4, 5, 6, 7, 8, 9

DEGREE OF ALLERGENIC SEVERITY: Occasional to moderate

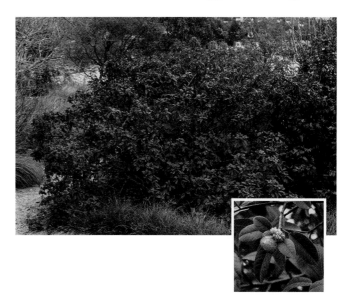

AREAS OF KNOWN PLANT

EXISTENCE:

Many of the buckthorn species are used as ornamental landscape plants; however, it is not a highly used plant and is only considered to be mildly "locally common" because of its lower population, even though its range of climate adaptability is quite broad. Naturally, the buckthorn grows on dry slopes, canyons and washes, pastures and roadsides, open woods, swamps and meadows, and is also an understory plant in mixed evergreen forested areas.

NATURAL CONCENTRATIONS:

Buckthorn species are found naturally in San Diego and San Bernadino Counties, and the Sierra Nevada Mountains from Placer County in California, northward to Washington. It grows along the California coastal chaparral sage and redwood forest. Also in northern Utah near streams and bogs at high elevations, Rocky Mountain region, northern Idaho, western Montana, southwest Colorado along streams and moist place on gravelly or sandy hills and flatlands at 7,000 feet elevation. Also on the northwest coast of Washington, Oregon and California, eastern central Arizona, spilling into western New Mexico.

In the East, buckthorn grows in southern Ohio, Illinois and West Virginia, North Dakota, south to northeast Kansas, east to North Carolina and into south and central Florida, extending west to central Texas, heading north into Missouri, and into North Dakota.

AREAS OF KNOWN ALLERGY

RELIEF:

Natural, unpopulated eastern Washington and Oregon. Central and northern Nevada, Wyoming, Atlantic Coast to Maine, Pennsylvania to Minnesota, and Oklahoma.

PARTIAL RELIEF:

Unpopulated areas of the Western states east of the Rocky Mountains, central Utah, central Idaho. Its ornamental use makes it hard to determine relief areas. Not an overly used plant in the landscape.

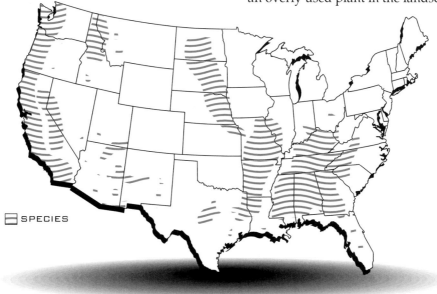

SPECIES

MONTHS OF ALLERGENIC SEVERITY

| JAN | FEB | MAR | APR | MAY | JNE | JLY | AUG | SEPT | OCT | NOV | DEC |

Allergy Producing Trees

■ BOTANICAL NAME: *Salix spp.*
COMMON NAME: **WILLOW**
USDA ZONES: 2, 3, 4, 5, 6, 7, 8

DEGREE OF ALLERGENIC SEVERITY: Occasional

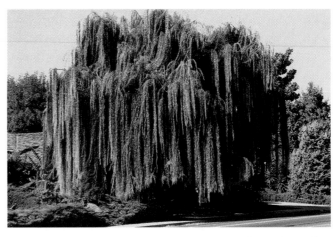

AREAS OF KNOWN PLANT

EXISTENCE:
There are many species of willow trees. They are widely planted in the United States, and should be considered "locally common" almost anywhere you find people. In the wild, willows grow in wet bogs to moist soils, near streams and in valley floors often associated with cottonwoods, black spruce, paper birch, oaks, junipers and pines. Some varieties of willow grow in dry desert areas, along beaches and coastal areas. Willows are found at almost all elevations below 11,000 feet.

NATURAL CONCENTRATIONS:
Willows can be found growing naturally along water courses throughout the Sierra Nevada Mountains and in southern California, along the Colorado River, in southern Arizona, northern New Mexico, and along some of the water courses in southern New Mexico and western Texas (El Paso area). Willows can also be found in the eastern part of Washington and along the Willamette and Umpqua Rivers, Oregon border on into the central and eastern portions of Idaho and in the Yellow Stone National Park in Wyoming. Willows are quite common east of the Rocky Mountains and throughout eastern Montana south to Wyoming.
In the East, willows are found throughout the states and Canada. A few specific areas include the valley of Wichita River in Oklahoma, Norfork County in Virginia, up the Savana River to Augusta in Georgia, near Apalachicola in Florida, near the shores of Lake Erie, central Missouri, New Orleans area, Louisiana, banks of the Potomac River, West Virginia, Turtle Mountains in North Dakota, Black Hills in South Dakota, and western Iowa.

AREAS OF KNOWN ALLERGY

RELIEF:
Unknown because it is widely planted as an ornamental and has a large distribution.

PARTIAL RELIEF:
Parts of unpopulated Nevada, central Oregon, Washington and southern Texas.

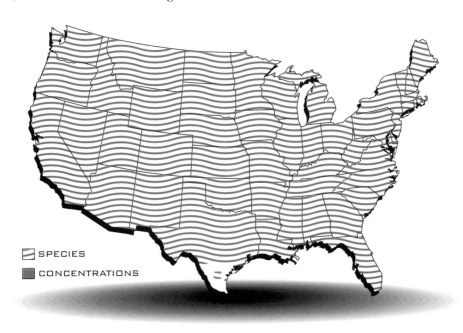

SPECIES
CONCENTRATIONS

MONTHS OF ALLERGENIC SEVERITY

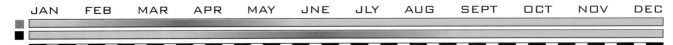

| JAN | FEB | MAR | APR | MAY | JNE | JLY | AUG | SEPT | OCT | NOV | DEC |

■ WESTERN STATES ■ EASTERN STATES

◤ BOTANICAL NAME: *Schinus molle*
COMMON NAME: **CALIFORNIA PEPPER**
USDA ZONES: 9, 10

DEGREE OF ALLERGENIC SEVERITY: Occasional

AREAS OF KNOWN PLANT

EXISTENCE:
The California pepper tree is actually native to South America and is used in the United States strictly as an ornamental landscape tree, so consider it moderately "locally common" within its USDA climate zones.

CONCENTRATIONS:
California pepper tree is found in cities, towns and populated areas within its USDA climate zones in California, Arizona, Texas, and Florida. It has escaped cultivation and is naturalizing in California and extreme southern Texas. California pepper is frost sensitive so it will not be found in the cold regions in the Midwest and East.

AREAS OF KNOWN ALLERGY

RELIEF:
USDA zones 1, 2, 3, 4, 5, 6. Natural unpopulated areas in the West. Central northern parts of the Midwest and East.

PARTIAL RELIEF:
Natural areas bordering populated areas, except Southern California and San Diego.

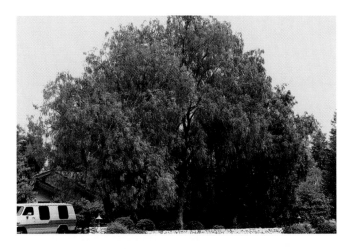

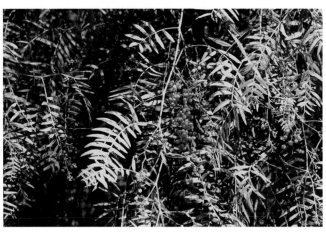

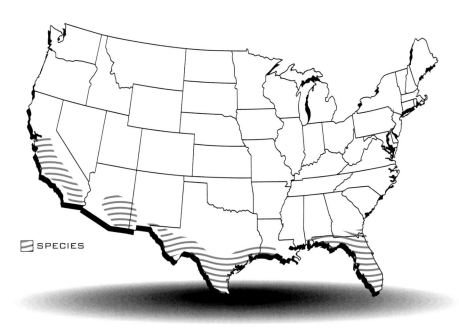

SPECIES

MONTHS OF ALLERGENIC SEVERITY

| JAN | FEB | MAR | APR | MAY | JNE | JLY | AUG | SEPT | OCT | NOV | DEC |

BOTANICAL NAME: *Tamarix spp.*
COMMON NAME: TAMARISK
USDA ZONES: 5, 6, 7, 8, 9

DEGREE OF ALLERGENIC SEVERITY: Moderate

AREAS OF KNOWN PLANT

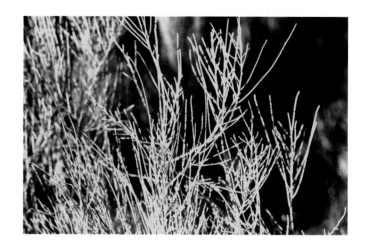

EXISTENCE:

The tamarisk tree/shrub is an introduced plant from southern Europe which has naturalized itself in the dry saline or along streams and boggy areas of the Southwest. Tamarix is also considered a "locally common" plant of minor importance except in areas of high concentrations as in the Southwest and southern California deserts.

NATURAL CONCENTRATIONS:

The tamarisk has taken hold in the Southwest and has spread and concentrated in many areas including the Great Salt Lake and Utah lake in Utah, along the Colorado River, Green River, Walker Lake, and in the Great Basin of Nevada and Utah and south Texas. Also the tamarisk can be found in San Diego and San Bernardino counties in California. The tamarisk is often found below 4,000 feet and is used as a wind break.

In the Midwest and East, tamarisk has spread into southwest Nebraska. It is reported to be spreading into Missouri, Kansas and escaping cultivation in Massachusetts and Indiana. It is reported to be used in the southeast as a sand dune stabilizer.

AREAS OF KNOWN ALLERGY

RELIEF:

Oregon, Washington, Idaho, Montana, and Wyoming. USDA zones 1, 2, 3, 4. Used as an ornamental tree/shrub so relief may be hard to identify.

PARTIAL RELIEF:

Elevations above 5,000 feet.

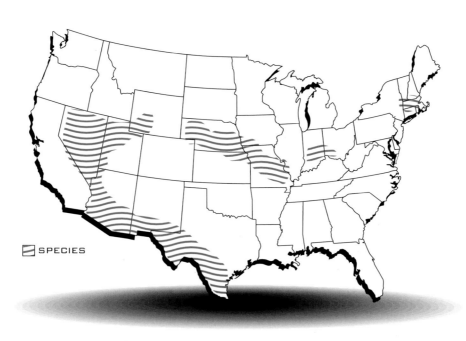

▱ SPECIES

MONTHS OF ALLERGENIC SEVERITY

| JAN | FEB | MAR | APR | MAY | JNE | JLY | AUG | SEPT | OCT | NOV | DEC |

BOTANICAL NAME: *Thuja occidentalis*
COMMON NAME: ARBOR-VITAE
USDA ZONES: 2, 3, 4, 5, 6, 7, 8

DEGREE OF ALLERGENIC SEVERITY: Occasional

AREAS OF KNOWN PLANT

EXISTENCE:
Arbor-vitae is an ornamental shrub and is considered "locally common" throughout its USDA zones. Naturally, arbor-vitae grows in swamps and cool, rocky banks. Other Thuja species are native to the Western United States

NATURAL CONCENTRATIONS:
Naturally arbor-vitae grows from Canada to Nova Scotia, North Carolina, Tennessee, Ohio, north Indiana, Wisconsin, Minnesota and northeast Illinois. Arbor-vitaes are concentrated in cities and towns in many areas across the United States. Concentrations of this plant are hard to determine; however, it is a popular landscape shrub and will likely be found in moderation throughout the populated areas within its USDA zones.

AREAS OF KNOWN ALLERGY

RELIEF:
Native or unpopulated areas of the West and Midwest, and natural desert areas.

PARTIAL RELIEF:
Iowa, and southern Minnesota.

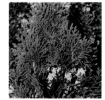

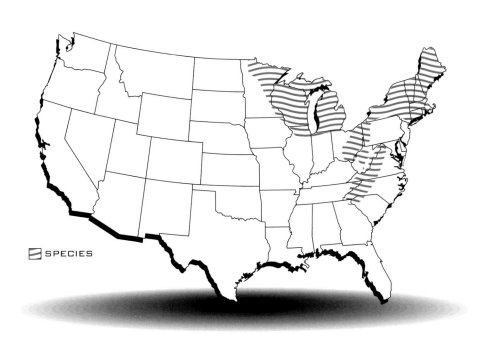

SPECIES

MONTHS OF ALLERGENIC SEVERITY

JAN   FEB   MAR   APR   MAY   JNE   JLY   AUG   SEPT   OCT   NOV   DEC

Allergy Producing Trees

BOTANICAL NAME: *Thuja plicata*
COMMON NAME: **WESTERN RED-CEDAR**
USDA ZONES: 5, 6, 7, 8

DEGREE OF ALLERGENIC SEVERITY: Moderate

AREAS OF KNOWN PLANT

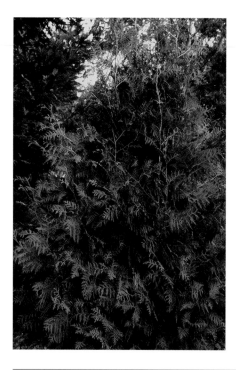

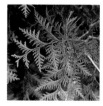

EXISTENCE:
The western red-cedar is a little less known as an ornamental or landscape tree, but it still manages to be seen in urban landscapes, so consider it to be "locally common" but to a lesser degree. Naturally, the western red-cedar grows in areas of moist, slightly acidic soil in association with other conifers and hemlock.

NATURAL CONCENTRATIONS:
Naturally western red-cedar can be found growing along the northern coast of California, Washington and Oregon and inland in northern Idaho and northwestern Montana at elevations of 3,000 feet in the north and 7,000 feet in the south.
In the East, western red-cedar is used as an ornamental and grows in many areas, including the Mid to North Atlantic states and as far north as Massachusetts.

AREAS OF KNOWN ALLERGY

RELIEF:
USDA zones 1, 2, 3, 4. Unpopulated areas of Arizona, New Mexico, Nevada, Utah, Colorado, southern half of the Gulf States from Texas to Florida, and Eastern states. Note that other species of (*Thuja*) red cedar have been suspected to cause allergies which may or may not grow in these areas of relief.

PARTIAL RELIEF:
Unpopulated areas of Central Oregon and Washington, southern Idaho, central and eastern Montana, and Midwest states.

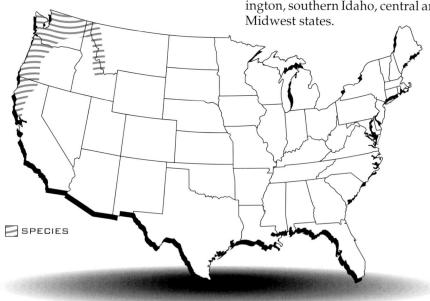

SPECIES

MONTHS OF ALLERGENIC SEVERITY

| JAN | FEB | MAR | APR | MAY | JNE | JLY | AUG | SEPT | OCT | NOV | DEC |

BOTANICAL NAME: *Ulmus spp.*
COMMON NAME: ELM
USDA ZONES: 2, 3, 4, 5, 6, 7, 8, 9

DEGREE OF ALLERGENIC SEVERITY: Moderate to high

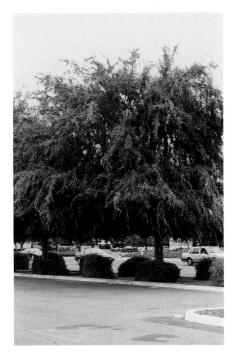
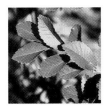

AREAS OF KNOWN PLANT

EXISTENCE:
Elms are not native to the West. Some are native to the Eastern United States and several of these have made their way out West as ornamental landscape trees. Consider elms highly "locally common" throughout the United States. Probably one of the most widely planted trees in the United States. Traveling through the United States, you'll find elm trees growing in every state and in most cities, towns, and rural areas. Elms like a variety of soils. Elms grow naturally in river bottom lands, low rich hills, banks and streams or in gravely dry uplands, and clay soils.

NATURAL CONCENTRATIONS:
Cities, towns, farms, and populated areas throughout. Elms are planted in high concentrations in the populated desert communities and outlying areas in the West. It is one of the toughest introduced landscape trees and survives well in the desert with minimal care.

In the East, elms grow naturally and are used ornamentally, or have spread from cultivation in all Midwest and Eastern states. A few specific areas include southern Kentucky, Valley of the Arkansas River, eastern Oklahoma near Muskogee County, St. Lawrence River Valley in Canada, Valley of the Sunflower River in Mississippi, Leon Rivers in Texas, western and central Florida near Lake Istokpoga, southeastern Virginia, southwestern Indiana, southern Illinois, southern Missouri, southern Ohio near Columbus, Michigan peninsula, central Wisconsin south to central and eastern Kansas, and Turtle Mountains in North Dakota.

AREAS OF KNOWN ALLERGY

RELIEF:
Natural unpopulated areas in the West, and in southern Florida.

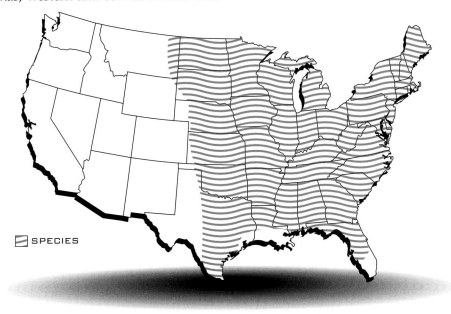

SPECIES

MONTHS OF ALLERGENIC SEVERITY

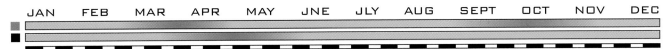

JAN FEB MAR APR MAY JNE JLY AUG SEPT OCT NOV DEC

■ WESTERN STATES ■ EASTERN STATES

BOTANICAL NAME: *Amaranthus spp.*
COMMON NAME: **PIGWEED,**
REDROOT PIG WEED,
PROSTRATE PIGWEED

DEGREE OF ALLERGENIC SEVERITY: High

AREAS OF KNOWN PLANT

EXISTENCE:
The pigweed species is very widespread and can be found throughout most of the United States and is considered a "locally common" weed. Pigweed has adapted to many types of soils and climate variations and can be found in cultivated fields, waste lands, gardens, landscapes, open lots, pastures, cracks and crevices in asphalt and concrete and roadsides. It's also related to the ornamental flowering cock's comb plant.

NATURAL CONCENTRATIONS:
Pigweed species can be found in abundance in low elevations of interior valleys in central and southern California, Antelope Valley, and Los Angeles County in California, as well as Phoenix, Flagstaff, Williams and Salt River Valley in Arizona, and Gallup in New Mexico. Areas in Montana, Oregon, eastern Washington, Colorado, and Mojave Deserts to Utah and Nevada near Soda Springs, Nevada County in Neveda. Most species of pigweed grow below 5,000 feet in elevation; however, *Amaranthus californicus* can reach elevations of 8,000 feet.
In the East, pigweed grows throughout the states including New England west to Missouri, and Kansas, Iowa, Michigan, south to Virginia. Less known in the Southern states, and in Florida.

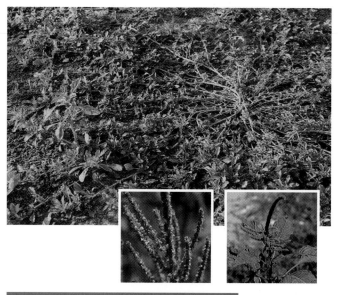

AREAS OF KNOWN ALLERGY

RELIEF:
Dry, arid, and non-irrigated and undisturbed soils.

PARTIAL RELIEF:
Elevations above 5,000 or 8,000 feet.

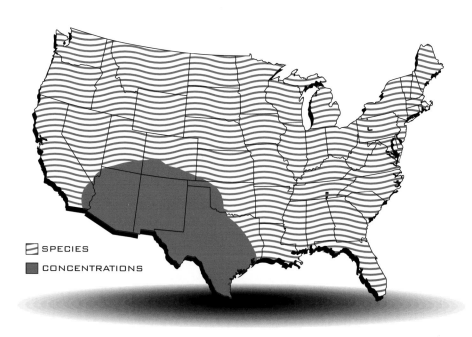

SPECIES
CONCENTRATIONS

MONTHS OF ALLERGENIC SEVERITY

JAN	FEB	MAR	APR	MAY	JNE	JLY	AUG	SEPT	OCT	NOV	DEC

BOTANICAL NAME: *Ambrosia spp.*
COMMON NAME: **SHORT, TALL, GIANT RAGWEED, WESTERN RAGWEED**

DEGREE OF ALLERGENIC SEVERITY: High

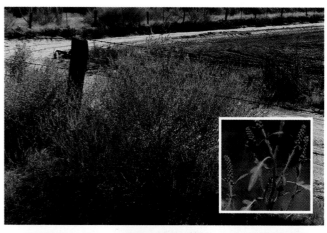

AREAS OF KNOWN PLANT

EXISTENCE:
Ragweed grows throughout the United States and should be considered "locally common" almost everywhere. Ragweed grows in a wide variety of soils; however, it is not very competitive and can be found growing in areas of low plant populations, i.e., ditches, road sides, wastelands, and open lots and fields.

NATURAL CONCENTRATIONS:
Ragweed can be found in concentrations in the following areas: California in Monterey, Santa Barbara, Orange, and San Joaquin counties, California foothills and coastal valleys, Lake Hodges to National City. Clark, Lincoln, and Nye counties in southern Nevada and into southern Utah. Southern Yuma County in Arizona. Also in Arizona mountains of Castle Dome, Gila, Cabeza Prietta, Tule and Mowhawk. Yellowstone National Forest area in Wyoming, and eastern Washington. Ragweed is also found in the Sonora desert to Durango, Colorado desert northward and along the Colorado River. Generally, ragweed grow between sea level and 3,000 feet in elevation.

In the East, at least one species of ragweed can be found in every state. Some states like Florida, Maine, northern Michigan, Wisconsin and northeastern Minnesota have only one dominant ragweed (*Ambrosia*) species. States with concentrated species or multiple species of rag-

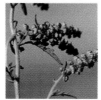
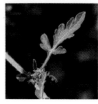
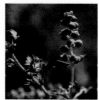

weed include Pennsylvania, west to eastern South Dakota, southeast North Dakota, southwestern Minnesota, eastern Nebraska, Kansas, Oklahoma and Texas, and east to the Atlantic states.

AREAS OF KNOWN ALLERGY

RELIEF:
Unknown.

PARTIAL RELIEF:
Washington and Oregon west of the Cascade Mountains. Higher elevations above 3,000 feet. Extreme northeastern Minnesota, northern Wisconsin, and northern Maine.

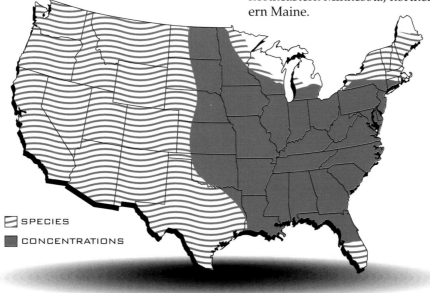

▨ SPECIES

▦ CONCENTRATIONS

MONTHS OF ALLERGENIC SEVERITY

| JAN | FEB | MAR | APR | MAY | JNE | JLY | AUG | SEPT | OCT | NOV | DEC |

BOTANICAL NAME: *Avena fatua*
COMMON NAME: WILD OAT

DEGREE OF ALLERGENIC SEVERITY: Moderate, higher in concentrations

AREAS OF KNOWN PLANT

EXISTENCE:
Since its introduction into the United States, the wild oat species has established throughout the Western states and most of the Eastern states. Considered to be "locally common" almost everywhere it grows. Wild oats grow in a wide variety of soils and can be found in pastures, open fields and lots, waste lands, road sides, fallow land, ditches, gardens, grain fields and agricultural crops, and railroad tracks. The cultivated oat is not considered to be allergenic because it is self-pollinated.

NATURAL CONCENTRATIONS:
The wild oat is found to be in higher concentrations in the Pacific states of California, western Oregon and Washington where it is reportedly more of a cause of allergies than elsewhere.
In the East, wild oats grow from Canada south to New England, Pennsylvania, Tennessee, Missouri, west to New Mexico, southeastern Texas, and are concentrated in Montana, North Dakota, and northern Minnesota. Wild oat is not as abundant elsewhere and consequently not an important cause of allergies.

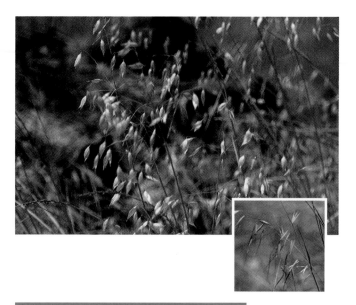

AREAS OF KNOWN ALLERGY

RELIEF:
Atlantic Coast to New Jersey, Gulf Coast states to southern Alabama and Louisiana, south and eastern Nebraska, Kansas, north, central, and western Texas.

PARTIAL RELIEF:
Higher elevations. Western, non-Pacific Coast States, central Arkansas, central Nebraska.

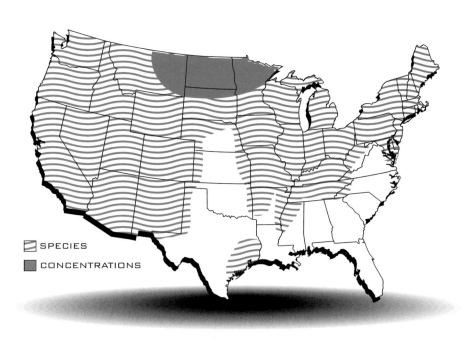

SPECIES
CONCENTRATIONS

MONTHS OF ALLERGENIC SEVERITY

JAN	FEB	MAR	APR	MAY	JNE	JLY	AUG	SEPT	OCT	NOV	DEC

WESTERN STATES   PACIFIC COAST

BOTANICAL NAME: *Bromus spp.*
COMMON NAME: BROME GRASS

DEGREE OF ALLERGENIC SEVERITY: Moderate, higher in Pacific States

AREAS OF KNOWN PLANT

EXISTENCE:

Brome grass has a wide range of flowering times depending on the region it is growing in. Brome grows below 10,500 feet in elevation and can be found growing in open ground, wastelands, and woodlands, especially at lower and middle elevations. Rarely found in dry, open places. Doesn't do well in dense shade.

NATURAL CONCENTRATIONS:

Brome grass can be found growing from British Columbia in Canada, south along the Pacific Coast and in Montana to New Mexico. Brome grass has been spotted growing in Arizona, and in the San Joaquin Valley and San Francisco in California.

In the East, brome grass grows in one species or another in every state. Higher concentrations exist in interior eastern states of Kentucky, Tennessee, Arkansas, northern Mississippi, Alabama and Louisiana, southern Missouri, Illinois, Indiana, Ohio, and West Virginia. Brome grass is more abundant on the West Coast, except in the Mideastern states, and consequently more of an allergy problem than elsewhere.

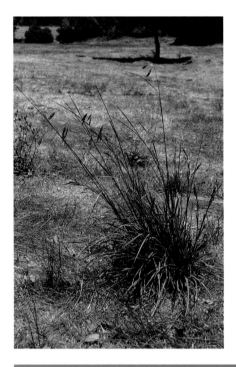
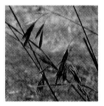

AREAS OF KNOWN ALLERGY

RELIEF:

Elevations above 10,500 feet. Dry and natural places.

PARTIAL RELIEF:

Dense, shaded wooded areas, southern Florida, northern Maine, between Lake Superior, Michigan, and the Rocky Mountains.

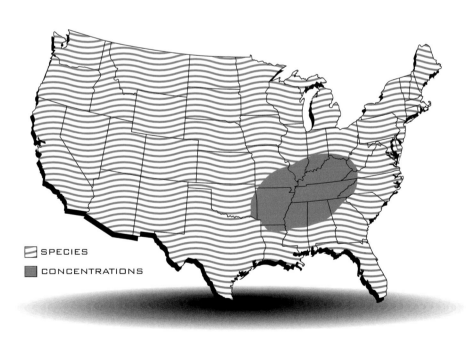

□ SPECIES
■ CONCENTRATIONS

MONTHS OF ALLERGENIC SEVERITY

| JAN | FEB | MAR | APR | MAY | JNE | JLY | AUG | SEPT | OCT | NOV | DEC |

BOTANICAL NAME: *Chenopodium spp.*
COMMON NAME: **LAMB'S-QUARTERS**

DEGREE OF ALLERGENIC SEVERITY: Moderate to high

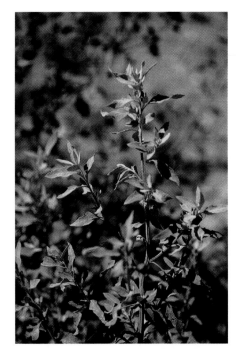

AREAS OF KNOWN PLANT

EXISTENCE:
There are many varieties of lamb's-quarters which have established themselves throughout the United States. The most recognized species are common lambsquarters (*Chenopodium album*) and Mexican tea (*Chenopodium ambrosioides*). Consider lamb's-quarters to be "locally common" in most areas. Lamb's-quarters grows best in areas of disturbed soil including cultivated fields, roadsides, pastures, vacant lots, fallow land, along streams, and near salt marshes.

NATURAL CONCENTRATIONS:
Lamb's-quarters is reported to cause allergy problems in Salt Lake City in Utah and is also located in Tucson, Phoenix, and Flagstaff in Arizona, and Gallup in New Mexico. Lamb's-quarters is also found in Pikes Peak and Colorado Springs in Colorado. An occasional weed in Washington and Oregon. Its highest western concentration appears to be in California.
In the East, lamb's-quarters grow extensively throughout all states. Concentrations occur from North Dakota east to Maryland and south to northern Florida and west to eastern Texas, with the highest concentration in the Mid-Atlantic states, and Southern states.

AREAS OF KNOWN ALLERGY

RELIEF:
Unknown.

PARTIAL RELIEF:
High elevations above 6,000 feet. Hot, dry uncultivated areas, parts of Washington, Oregon, and Neveda.

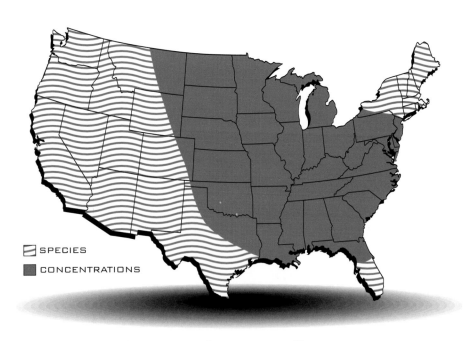

SPECIES
CONCENTRATIONS

MONTHS OF ALLERGENIC SEVERITY

| JAN | FEB | MAR | APR | MAY | JNE | JLY | AUG | SEPT | OCT | NOV | DEC |

BOTANICAL NAME: *Cynodon dactylon*
COMMON NAME: BERMUDA GRASS

DEGREE OF ALLERGENIC SEVERITY: Very high

AREAS OF KNOWN PLANT

EXISTENCE:
Bermuda grass can be found growing aggressively in warmer temperate regions in the United States. Bermuda grass is used primarily as a pasture and lawn grass. It has escaped to areas such as roadsides, agricultural ground, open fields, vacant lots, unkempt areas, and railroad tracks.

CONCENTRATIONS:
Bermuda grass is a universal grass in California, Oregon, Arizona, New Mexico, and southern and central Utah. It is found in other colder climate states but is not as aggressive or abundant. Bermuda grass is one of the worst allergy offenders. It has been reported to be a major allergy factor in Tucson in Arizona. In fact, Tucson has such a bad allergy problem from pollen that they passed an ordinance against certain allergy causing plants. In the Southwestern states bermuda grass can pollinate from late January to early December. In Northwestern states it is limited to the late spring, summer and early fall periods.

In the East, bermuda grass is concentrated mostly in the Southern states and north to northern Kentucky, southern Indiana and Illinois. Bermuda grows in other states to a lesser aggressive degree from Kansas east through Missouri, northern Illinois, Indiana and Ohio, Pennsylvania, to southern New Hampshire.

AREAS OF KNOWN ALLERGY

RELIEF:
Natural cold climate areas. Natural, arid areas of little or no summer water (medium to high deserts). Michigan to Montana, and south to Nebraska. Northern Vermont and New Hampshire, and Maine.

PARTIAL RELIEF:
Natural or less populated areas of Nevada, Wyoming, Montana, Colorado, Appalachian Mountains, and northern New York.

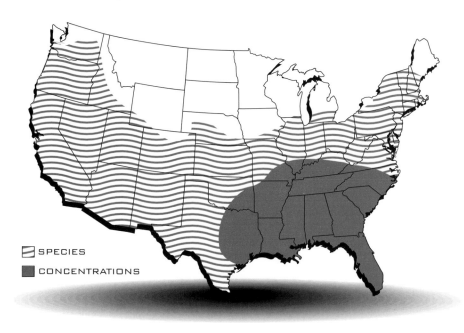

SPECIES
CONCENTRATIONS

MONTHS OF ALLERGENIC SEVERITY

| JAN | FEB | MAR | APR | MAY | JNE | JLY | AUG | SEPT | OCT | NOV | DEC |

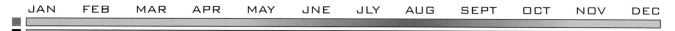

■ WARM WINTER AREAS

Allergy Producing Weeds and Grasses

BOTANICAL NAME: *Dactylis glomerata*
COMMON NAME: **ORCHARD GRASS,**
COCK'S-FOOT GRASS

DEGREE OF ALLERGENIC SEVERITY: High

AREAS OF KNOWN PLANT

EXISTENCE:
Orchard grass has escaped cultivation and can be found growing in wastelands, roadsides, moist meadows and lawns. Orchard grass is widely used as hay and is grown between the rows of orchard trees (hence the name orchard grass). In some areas in could be considered "locally common."

CONCENTRATIONS:
Orchard grass can be found almost throughout the Western United States.
In the East, orchard grass is found from Canada south to Alabama. Not much information exists on the specific location of this plant.

AREAS OF KNOWN ALLERGY

RELIEF:
Unknown.

PARTIAL RELIEF:
Hot, dry, sunny locations. Higher elevations in the Pacific Northwest, and Midwest states.

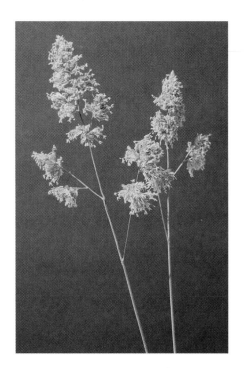

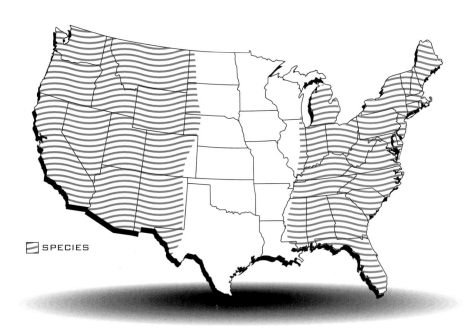

SPECIES

MONTHS OF ALLERGENIC SEVERITY

| JAN | FEB | MAR | APR | MAY | JNE | JLY | AUG | SEPT | OCT | NOV | DEC |

BOTANICAL NAME: *Holcus lanatus*
COMMON NAME: VELVET GRASS

DEGREE OF ALLERGENIC SEVERITY: Moderate to high in abundant amounts

AREAS OF KNOWN PLANT

EXISTENCE:
Velvet grass is generally found in cultivated fields, pastures, wetlands, waste areas and has escaped cultivation. Not much information has been published concerning this plant.

CONCENTRATIONS:
Velvet grass is found mostly in the Pacific Northwest and northern California below 7,500 feet in elevation, western Washington and Oregon, west of the Cascade Mountains, northern counties of Humbolt and Mendocino in California. It has been found growing in Idaho and Montana.
In the East, velvet grass is known to grow from Canada to Michigan, south to Georgia and Louisiana. Other areas are suspected.

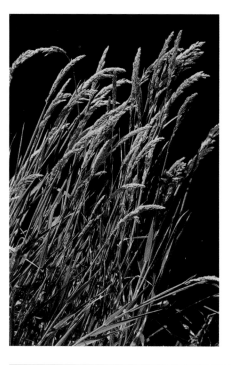

AREAS OF KNOWN ALLERGY

RELIEF:
Southern California, Nevada, eastern Washington and Oregon, Utah, Arizona, New Mexico, Colorado, Texas, Maine, and Midwest.

PARTIAL RELIEF:
Florida and elevations above 7,500 feet.

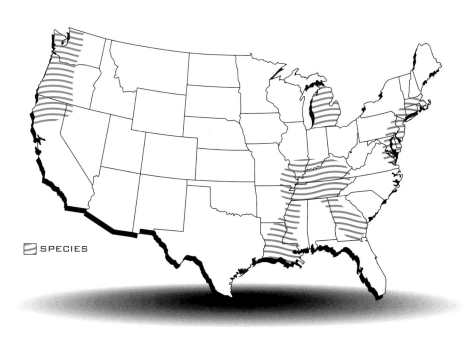

MONTHS OF ALLERGENIC SEVERITY

JAN FEB MAR APR MAY JNE JLY AUG SEPT OCT NOV DEC

BOTANICAL NAME: *Lolium spp.*
COMMON NAME: **RYEGRASS**

DEGREE OF ALLERGENIC SEVERITY: Moderate, high near Corvallis in Oregon

AREAS OF KNOWN PLANT

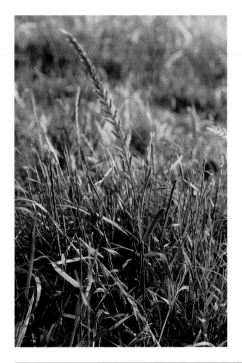

EXISTENCE:
Rye grass is mostly used as a short term lawn grass, in urban and rural settings especially where bermuda grass lawns are grown. Rye grass generally doesn't cause allergy problems if the flower spikes are mowed weekly. Rye grass is also used as a pasture grass. As a pasture grass it usually matures to form a flower spike in some areas within the pasture where grazing is overlooked. Rye grass has spread throughout the United States along roadsides, waste or idle lands, and in grain fields.

NATURAL CONCENTRATIONS:
Rye grass is grown for seed near Corvallis, Oregon. The grass is allowed to go to seed so the pollen concentration in and near Corvallis will be high during the pollination season. Naturally, rye grass is found growing along the Pacific States including California coast rangeland in and among oak woodland areas. Rye grass can be found throughout most of the United States, including, but certainly not limited to, Minnesota, Kansas, south to the Gulf Coast States, Delaware, and Washington D. C.

AREAS OF KNOWN ALLERGY

RELIEF:
Unknown. Possibly dry and unpopulated desert areas.

PARTIAL RELIEF:
Unknown.

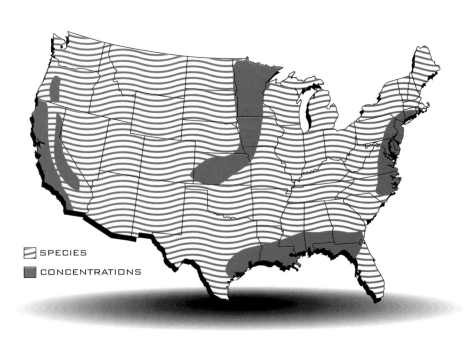

SPECIES

CONCENTRATIONS

MONTHS OF ALLERGENIC SEVERITY

| JAN | FEB | MAR | APR | MAY | JNE | JLY | AUG | SEPT | OCT | NOV | DEC |

BOTANICAL NAME: *Plantago lanceolata*
COMMON NAME: ENGLISH PLANTAIN, BUCKHORN

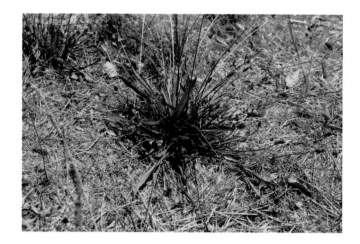

DEGREE OF ALLERGENIC SEVERITY: Moderate, high in concentrations

AREAS OF KNOWN PLANT

EXISTENCE:
English plantain has naturalized in both idle and cultivated fields, roadsides, lawns, waste places, and grasslands throughout the United States. English plantain has truly become a cosmopolitan weed. It is found in rural and urban areas.

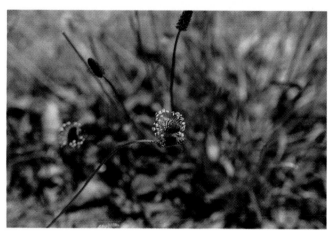

NATURAL CONCENTRATIONS:
English plantain can be found in intermountain valleys of western Montana and central Idaho. It is found in California and west of the Cascade mountains in Oregon and Washington and in sandy desert hillsides of Utah.

In the East, English plantain grows in most states and is concentrated from Missouri to New Jersey, south to North Carolina, Tennessee, and northern Arkansas.

AREAS OF KNOWN ALLERGY

RELIEF:
Unknown

PARTIAL RELIEF:
Natural, non-irrigated or dry areas, and uncultivated areas.

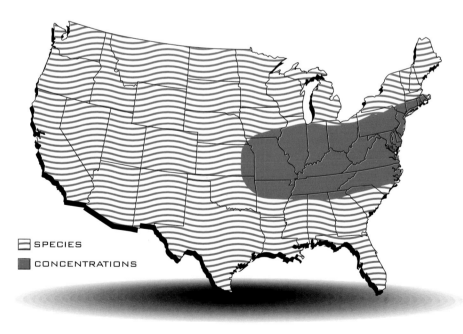

□ SPECIES
■ CONCENTRATIONS

MONTHS OF ALLERGENIC SEVERITY

| JAN | FEB | MAR | APR | MAY | JNE | JLY | AUG | SEPT | OCT | NOV | DEC |

Allergy Producing Weeds and Grasses

■ BOTANICAL NAME: *Rumex acetosella*
COMMON NAME: **SORREL,**
DOCK

DEGREE OF ALLERGENIC SEVERITY: Moderate, high
in concentrations

AREAS OF KNOWN PLANT

EXISTENCE:
Sorrel is found in pastures, wastelands, lawns,
roadsides, gardens, areas of poor drainage and in soils
low in fertility. Sometimes an indicator of acidic soils, although sorrel will grow in neutral and alkaline soils, especially if the nitrogen levels are low. Often associated
with cultivated soils, agriculture land, and developments.

NATURAL CONCENTRATIONS:
Sorrel is widespread, growing from Canada,
southwest through California and east through Colorado,
to the East Coast and many places in between. Sorrel is
found concentrated in northern California and north to
Washington.
In the East, from Missouri to Pennsylvania, south
to northern North Carolina, Tennessee, and Arkansas.

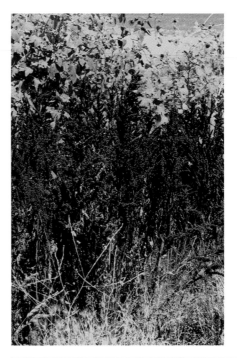

AREAS OF KNOWN ALLERGY

RELIEF:
Unknown

PARTIAL RELIEF:
Natural and dry desert areas of the West.

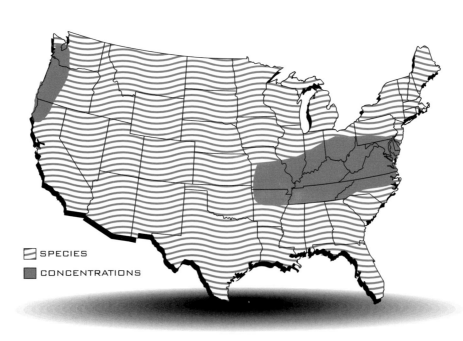

SPECIES

CONCENTRATIONS

MONTHS OF ALLERGENIC SEVERITY

| JAN | FEB | MAR | APR | MAY | JNE | JLY | AUG | SEPT | OCT | NOV | DEC |

BOTANICAL NAME: *Salsola kali*
COMMON NAME: **RUSSIAN THISTLE, TUMBLEWEED**

DEGREE OF ALLERGENIC SEVERITY: Moderate to high

AREAS OF KNOWN PLANT

EXISTENCE:

The Russian thistle or tumbleweed is quite established in the West, Midwest, Gulf Coast and Atlantic coastal areas. It is found along roadsides, cultivated fields or areas of disturbed soil, open lots, fallow land, and waste areas. It is very tolerant of alkaline soils and is very common in many western deserts. This plant should be considered "locally common" especially in drier, arid areas often in association with over grazed areas.

NATURAL CONCENTRATIONS:

Russian thistle is found in the Chiuhauhua Desert in northern Arizona, and New Mexico, throughout most of the Rocky Mountains and Great Basin areas. Also in Wyoming and Utah, below the eastern slope of the Sierra Nevada forest in California, northern California north to western Washington, and parts of eastern Washington and Oregon. It is concentrated from North Dakota south to central and southern Texas. Russian thistle is generally found at elevations below 3,500 feet.

In the East, Russian thistle is generally confined to the southern parts of the Gulf Coast States along the eastern parts of the Atlantic states to Maine.

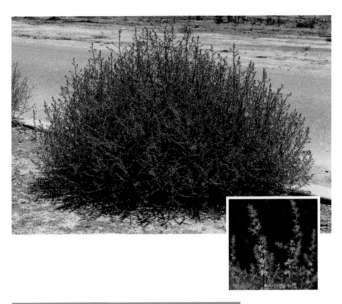

AREAS OF KNOWN ALLERGY

RELIEF:

High elevations above 4,000 feet in semitropical areas, northern parts of the Gulf states to Wisconsin, east to New York.

PARTIAL RELIEF:

High elevation forested area, eastern Minnesota, Iowa and Missouri, and northeastern Arkansas to western Virginia.

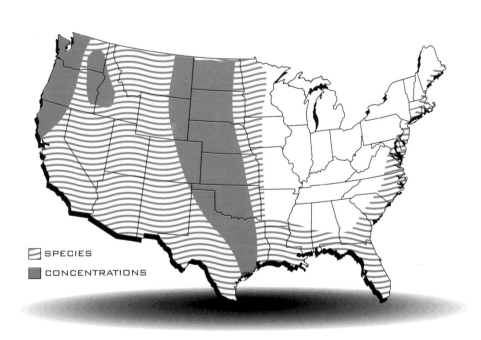

SPECIES
CONCENTRATIONS

MONTHS OF ALLERGENIC SEVERITY

| JAN | FEB | MAR | APR | MAY | JNE | JLY | AUG | SEPT | OCT | NOV | DEC |

BOTANICAL NAME: *Sorghum halepense*
COMMON NAME: JOHNSON GRASS

DEGREE OF ALLERGENIC SEVERITY: High

AREAS OF KNOWN PLANT

EXISTENCE:

Johnson grass was originally imported to the United States as a forage crop. It quickly escaped its boundaries to become one of the worst allergy causing grasses in the United States. Johnson grass is found growing along roadsides, ditches, agricultural land, vacant or open lots, fallow land, gardens and lawns, usually in warmer irrigated areas of the United States. Johnson grass is not as aggressive in colder climates, and thus not as great an allergy threat in these areas.

CONCENTRATIONS:

Johnson grass is quite abundant in the interior valleys in northern and southern California areas. As a general rule, wherever there is farming in California there is Johnson grass. Other areas of abundance of Johnson grass are the Dixie area and Northern Counties in Utah and irrigated areas of Arizona. Johnson grass is found in the central part of Oregon and Washington at the border.

Towards the East, Johnson grass grows south of northern Colorado through southern Michigan, and New York to central New Hampshire. Johnson grass is concentrated in the warmer climates from Southern Missouri, south to Florida, east to southern South Carolina, and west to eastern Texas.

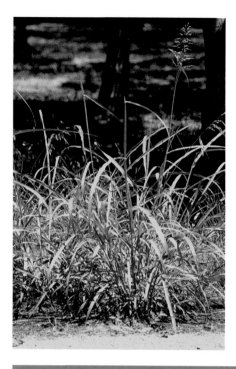
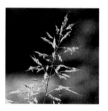

AREAS OF KNOWN ALLERGY

RELIEF:

Natural, unpopulated and non-farming areas of Montana, Idaho, Wyoming and Nevada, North and South Dakota, Minnesota, Wisconsin, central and northern Michigan, northern New York, northern Vermont, New Hampshire, and Maine.

PARTIAL RELIEF:

Central and northern California coast. Most areas of the Great Basin, northern Utah, Nebraska, Iowa. Colder, high elevation areas.

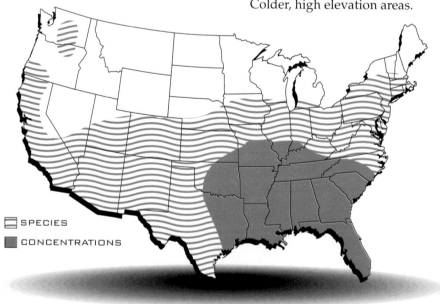

SPECIES
CONCENTRATIONS

MONTHS OF ALLERGENIC SEVERITY

| JAN | FEB | MAR | APR | MAY | JNE | JLY | AUG | SEPT | OCT | NOV | DEC |

BOTANICAL NAME: *Trifolium spp.*
COMMON NAME: CLOVER

DEGREE OF ALLERGENIC SEVERITY: Occasional, moderate in concentration

AREAS OF KNOWN PLANT

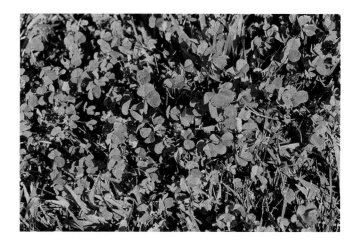

EXISTENCE:
 Clover grows throughout the United States with a higher concentration in the Pacific states and mountain desert regions. Naturally, clover grows in fields, pastures, roadsides, meadows, woods, and moist areas. Also clover is common in lawns and is grown as a cover or forage crop.

NATURAL CONCENTRATIONS:
 There are over 75 species of clover in the United States. Most of them are concentrated in the West primarily in California and Oregon.
 In the East, the number of clover species is less; however, their distribution is throughout. Some specific areas include Thompkins County in New York, Illinois, south to Kansas and Alabama, Prince Edwards County in Virginia, Florida to Texas.

AREAS OF KNOWN ALLERGY

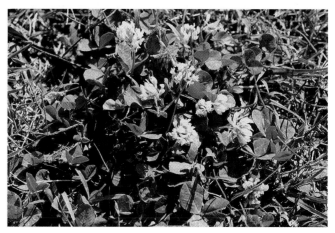

RELIEF:
 Unknown. Hard to establish relief because of it's native, ornamental, and agricultural uses.

PARTIAL RELIEF:
 Dry and unirrigated areas.

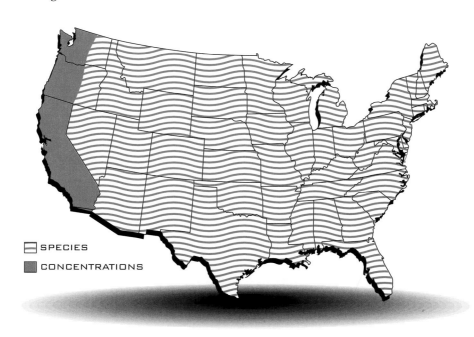

SPECIES
CONCENTRATIONS

MONTHS OF ALLERGENIC SEVERITY

JAN	FEB	MAR	APR	MAY	JNE	JLY	AUG	SEPT	OCT	NOV	DEC

Chapter 6   149

BOTANICAL NAME: *Xanthium spp.*
COMMON NAME: **COCKLEBUR**

DEGREE OF ALLERGENIC SEVERITY: Moderate to High

AREAS OF KNOWN PLANT

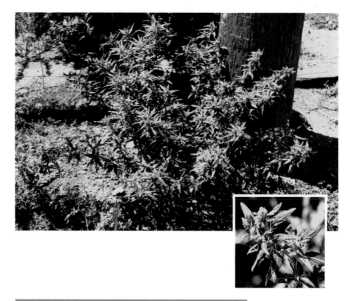

EXISTENCE:

The cocklebur has spread throughout most of the United States metropolitan areas to become quite the cosmopolitan plant. It is mildly considered "locally common" in warmer areas of lower elevations. Cocklebur can be found along ditches, pastures, and wetland areas, including exposed river, and lake bottoms, and adjacent areas. It can also be found in many intercity areas.

NATURAL CONCENTRATIONS:

Cocklebur is found in moist areas of valley floors in California, Kaweah Lake, San Francisco Bay area, and other lower foothill areas in California and the West. Cocklebur is found in areas were grazing stock (cows and sheep) frequent. The seed adheres to the fir of animals and is distributed as they migrate.

In the East, cocklebur grows to the Atlantic Coast and everywhere in between, except northern New York, Vermont, New Hampshire, and Maine. It is concentrated from eastern Wyoming to Pennsylvania, south to northern Florida and west to central Texas and states in between.

AREAS OF KNOWN ALLERGY

RELIEF:

Higher elevations in cold areas of the West, northern New Hampshire and Vermont, and Maine.

PARTIAL RELIEF:

Dry, arid, and non-irrigated areas.

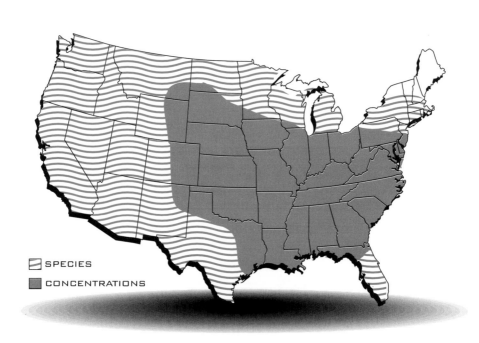

SPECIES

CONCENTRATIONS

MONTHS OF ALLERGENIC SEVERITY

JAN	FEB	MAR	APR	MAY	JNE	JLY	AUG	SEPT	OCT	NOV	DEC

WESTERN STATES ■ EASTERN STATES

BOTANICAL NAME: *Amaranthus spp.*
COMMON NAME: **AMARANTHUS**
USDA ZONES: 2, 3, 4, 5, 6, 7, 8, 9, 10, 11, annual

DEGREE OF ALLERGENIC SEVERITY: Occasional

AREAS OF KNOWN PLANT

EXISTENCE:
Ornamental amaranthus are mildly planted throughout the United States, almost entirely in urban and rural gardens. Consider them to be "locally common." They prefer poorer soils, and when planted in quantities can cause allergy symptoms.

CONCENTRATIONS:
Ornamental amarnthus can be found in land-scapes and gardens in many cities, towns and rural communities throughout the United States. Fortunately, they are not grown in great abundance.

AREAS OF KNOWN ALLERGY

RELIEF:
Relief from the family of amaranthus can be diffi-cult. The weedy cousin of the ornamental amaranthus (Pigweed) is widespread so relief can be difficult; how-ever, relief from the ornamental amaranthus can be ac-complished in natural, unpopulated areas in the United States.

PARTIAL RELIEF:
Try elevations above 5,000 or 8,000 feet.

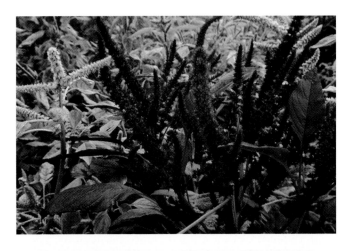

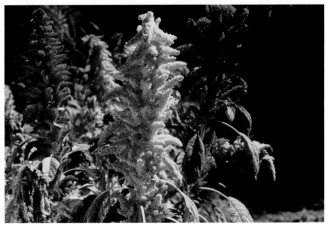

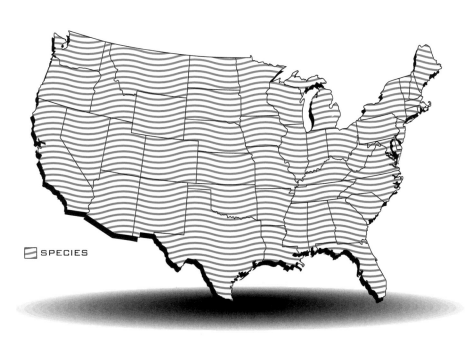

☐ SPECIES

MONTHS OF ALLERGENIC SEVERITY

| JAN | FEB | MAR | APR | MAY | JNE | JLY | AUG | SEPT | OCT | NOV | DEC |

BOTANICAL NAME: *Chrysanthemum spp.*
COMMON NAME: **MUMS, FEVERFEW, SHASTA DAISY, DUSTY MILLER**
USDA ZONES: 2, 3, 4, 5, 6, 7, 8, 9, 10, 11, annual

DEGREE OF ALLERGENIC SEVERITY: Occasional

AREAS OF KNOWN PLANT

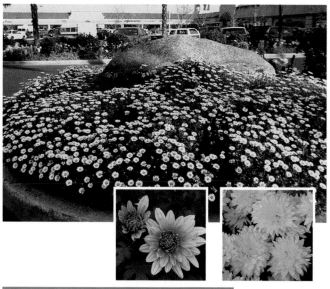

EXISTENCE:
There are several species of chrysanthemums from the typical florists' mum to the shasta daisy. In some cases the chrysanthemums have escaped cultivation and naturalized in the United States, particularly in California. Consider chrysanthemums to be "locally common" throughout the United States. Natural Chrysanthemums grow in gravelly or sandy soils, along streams or dry slopes, meadows and pastures.

NATURAL CONCENTRATIONS:
Chrysanthemums have escaped cultivation in the greater San Diego area and along the coastal areas of central and northern California. An occasional occurrence of wild chrysanthemum has been noted west of the Cascade Mountains in Oregon and Washington.

In the East chrysanthemum species can be found throughout, concentrating from eastern Minnesota then diagonally east to northern South Carolina, extending north to Maryland, Pennsylvania and to Wisconsin. Chrysanthemums or "mums" are often grown in pots and given as gifts intended for indoor enjoyment. However, mums indoors can increase the concentration and duration of exposure to the pollen, thus increasing the potential for allergy symptoms to occur in those sensitive to chrysanthemums.

AREAS OF KNOWN ALLERGY

RELIEF:
Natural non-populated areas of Wyoming, Montana, Colorado, Utah, Nevada, New Mexico, Idaho, and Arizona. Understand that chrysanthemums (as a floral arrangement) can be found indoors anywhere.

PARTIAL RELIEF:
Natural, unpopulated areas of inner, central and northern California and eastern Oregon and Washington, western Montana and Wyoming, North Dakota, and South Dakota.

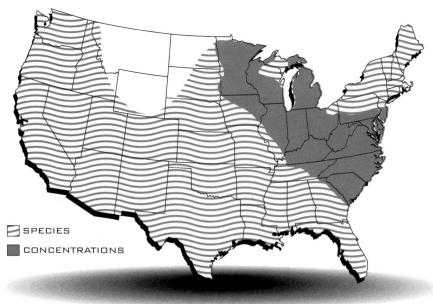

SPECIES
CONCENTRATIONS

MONTHS OF ALLERGENIC SEVERITY

| JAN | FEB | MAR | APR | MAY | JNE | JLY | AUG | SEPT | OCT | NOV | DEC |

BOTANICAL NAME: *Dahlia spp.*
COMMON NAME: **DAHLIA**
USDA ZONES: 2, 3, 4, 5, 6, 7, 8, 9, 10, 11, annual

DEGREE OF ALLERGENIC SEVERITY: Occasional

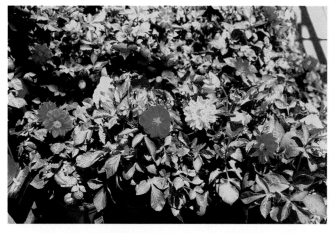

AREAS OF KNOWN PLANT

EXISTENCE:
Dahlias are grown strictly for their ornamental appeal and do not grow naturally in the United States. Consider them to be "locally common" in most urban and rural gardens.

CONCENTRATIONS:
There are no known areas where dahlias naturally exist in the United States. Even in cultivation we could not find areas of large concentrations of dahlias; however, they will be found scattered about with some consistency in city and rural gardens throughout the United States. Some dahlias are grown in pots and given as gifts intended for indoor enjoyment. However, dahlias indoors can increase the concentration and duration of exposure to pollen, thus increasing the potential for the allergy sufferer(s) to have allergy symptoms.

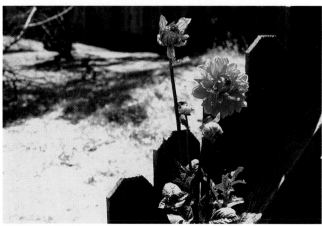

AREAS OF KNOWN ALLERGY

RELIEF:
Since dahlias are not native nor have they naturalized in the United States, relief should be found in areas of natural vegetation in unpopulated areas.

PARTIAL RELIEF:
Natural unpopulated areas.

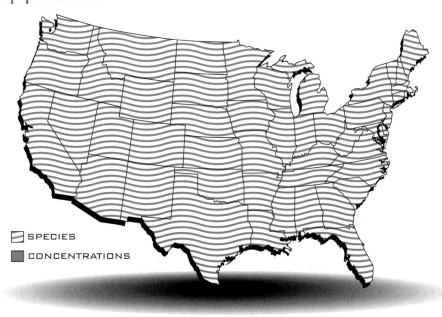

SPECIES

CONCENTRATIONS

MONTHS OF ALLERGENIC SEVERITY

JAN	FEB	MAR	APR	MAY	JNE	JLY	AUG	SEPT	OCT	NOV	DEC

Allergy Producing Flowers

■ BOTANICAL NAME: *Helianthus annuus*
COMMON NAME: **SUNFLOWER**
USDA ZONES: 2, 3, 4, 5, 6, 7, 8, 9, 10, 11, annual

DEGREE OF ALLERGENIC SEVERITY: Occasional to moderate

AREAS OF KNOWN PLANT

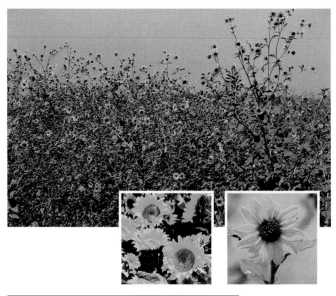

EXISTENCE:
There are two distinct sunflower plants. One grows wild (weedy shrub with many small 2" to 3" sunflowers) and the other is commercially grown for its seed, better known as "sunflower seeds" (single stem and one large flower). Sunflowers naturally grow along roadsides, fields, waste places, fence lines, open lots and lowland areas up to 5,000 feet.

NATURAL CONCENTRATIONS:
There is little information on the concentrations of the Sunflower in the United States. Most reports state that it is widespread throughout the United States. However, some information indicates that the sunflower can be found concentrated in open sandy desert areas of southern and eastern Utah and in the San Joaquin and Sacramento Valleys of California. Other concentrations are certain to exist.

In the East, sunflowers grow in their native states of Minnesota, south to Missouri, Texas, and Canada. Sunflowers grow in all other states and are also concentrated from South Dakota east to Connecticut, south to central Florida and west to eastern Texas, Oklahoma, Iowa, and Nebraska.

AREAS OF KNOWN ALLERGY

RELIEF:
Elevation above 5,000 feet.

PARTIAL RELIEF:
Northern coastal ranges and the Mojave desert in California.

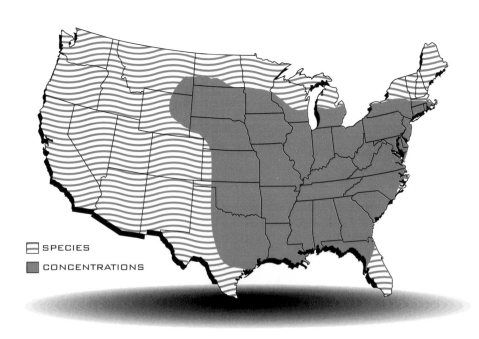

◧ SPECIES
■ CONCENTRATIONS

MONTHS OF ALLERGENIC SEVERITY

| JAN | FEB | MAR | APR | MAY | JNE | JLY | AUG | SEPT | OCT | NOV | DEC |

BOTANICAL NAME: *Rudbeckia hirta*
COMMON NAME: **BLACK-EYED SUSAN**

USDA ZONES: 2, 3, 4, 5, 6, 7, 8, 9, 10, 11, annual

DEGREE OF ALLERGENIC SEVERITY: Occasional

AREAS OF KNOWN PLANT

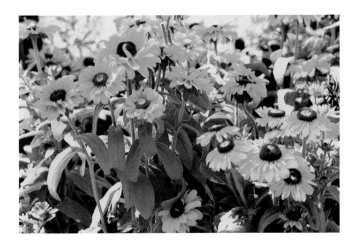

EXISTENCE:
Black-eyed Susans have been introduced to the West from the Eastern United States. They grow in a variety of situations, including mountain meadows, moist lowland or valleys and in disturbed soil. Black-eyed Susan is better known as an ornamental annual or short-lived perennial so consider them "locally common."

NATURAL CONCENTRATIONS:
Occasional naturalized concentrations of black-eyed Susan can be found in the middle altitude meadows of the Sierra Nevada Mountains in California from Amador County to Mariposa County, and occasionally in moist areas in the Central Valley. Mid-1930 reports found black-eyed Susan growing in Colorado. Other species of black-eyed Susan have been found from Montana to Arizona and New Mexico.

In the East, black-eyed-Susan is concentrated in western Massachusetts to Illinois, south to Georgia and Alabama. Other species are found throughout the United States. Black-eyed Susan is also an ornamental plant, so consider the concentrations to be higher in populated areas. Fortunately black-eyed Susans are not grown ornamentally in large numbers.

AREAS OF KNOWN ALLERGY

RELIEF:
Most likely relief can be found in unpopulated desert or dry areas in the West, Midwest, and Northeast.

PARTIAL RELIEF:
Unpopulated areas along the west coast. High altitude above 8,000 feet.

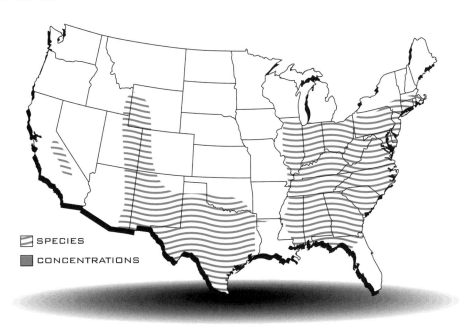

SPECIES
CONCENTRATIONS

MONTHS OF ALLERGENIC SEVERITY

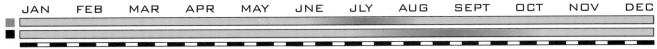

| JAN | FEB | MAR | APR | MAY | JNE | JLY | AUG | SEPT | OCT | NOV | DEC |

■ WESTERN STATES ■ EASTERN STATES

■ BOTANICAL NAME: *Zinnia spp.*
   COMMON NAME: **ZINNIA**

USDA ZONES: 1, 2, 3, 4, 5, 6, 7, 8, 9, 10, annual

DEGREE OF ALLERGENIC SEVERITY: Occasional

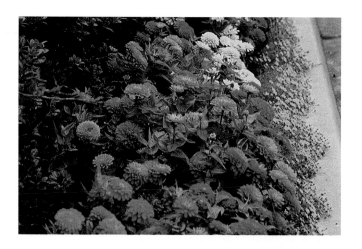

AREAS OF KNOWN PLANT

EXISTENCE:
   Zinnias have not escaped in any appreciable number into the wild. Therefore, zinnias are strictly limited to the populated areas of the United States. Zinnias are a very popular summer (annual) flower and should be considered very "locally common" throughout the United States except in areas of high summer moisture (they suffer from mildew).

CONCENTRATIONS:
   Zinnias' popularity seems to fluctuate from year to year. The increase or decrease in usage tends to follow a two to three year trend. The concentration of zinnias will be limited to the urban and rural areas.

AREAS OF KNOWN ALLERGY

RELIEF:
   Native unpopulated areas in the United States

PARTIAL RELIEF:
   Areas of high summer moisture and rural areas.

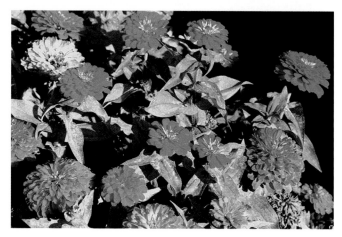

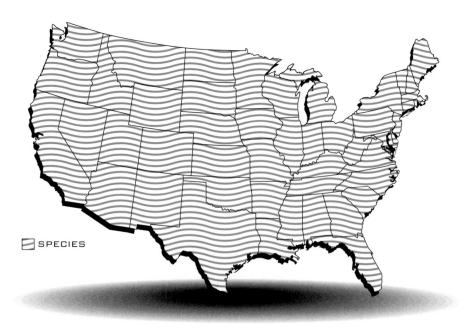

▨ SPECIES

MONTHS OF ALLERGENIC SEVERITY

| JAN | FEB | MAR | APR | MAY | JNE | JLY | AUG | SEPT | OCT | NOV | DEC |

Chapter 7

*P*hoto Illustrations Of Landscapes

◣ *Good and Bad Landscapes*

This chapter is dedicated to illustrating the good and bad landscape settings using photographs with written explanations. Examples of allergy-free landscapes allow the allergy sufferer to actually see allergy-free plantings and how they interact in the landscape. Using these examples as a guide will enable the allergy sufferer to successfully plan and implement the reconstruction of his or her landscape(s). As you look and read through the following chapter you will no doubt find combinations of plants that appeal to you. However, as you formulate a plant list for your own landscape make sure the plants you choose are compatible and are complimentary in theme, size, shape, color, texture, and water requirements. For example planting a yucca next to a redwood would be a violation of both the landscape theme and water usage. Yuccas would be more at home in a desert or western setting. On the other hand redwoods lean towards an alpine or woodsy setting. Furthermore, yuccas do not require much water once they are established and redwoods need consistent moisture. Examples of allergy producing landscapes are also provided to illustrate how and what not to plant. Study these examples and think of the plantings in your neighborhood landscapes, parks, and shopping complexes that resemble these and look for good allergy-free replacements (Chapter 8). Communicate your ideas to others in your community and start planting allergy-free plants, whenever feasible, in place of allergy producing plants. Educating the public, and the consistent planting of allergy-free plants while reducing and or eliminating non-essential allergy producing plants, will over time, significantly reduce the number and occurrences of allergy symptoms.

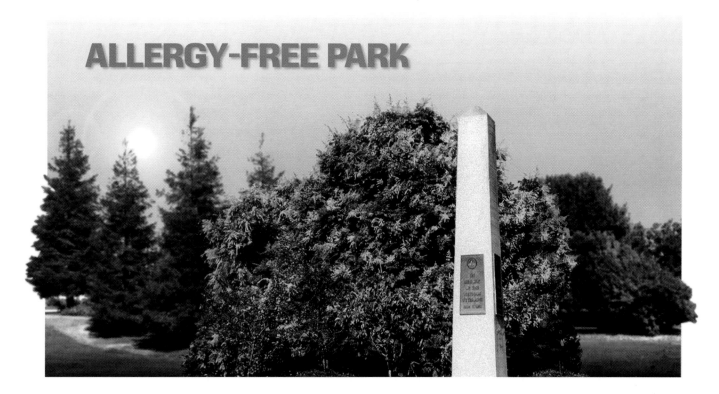

This parking lot is a good example of an allergy-free semipublic area. The trees are ornamental pears with golden shrub daisies and pansies underneath. Every little bit helps. No area is too small for allergy-free planting.

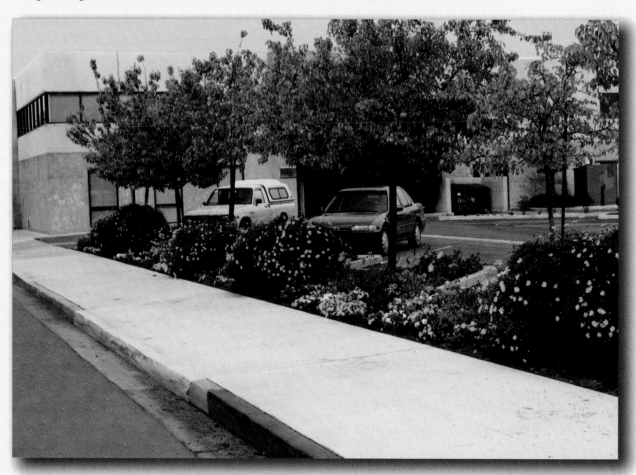

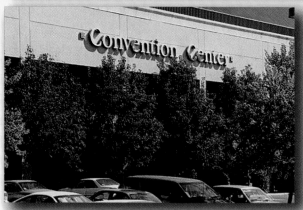

Some buildings are built with public funds. Our tax dollars shouldn't be spent on things that can make us sick or miserable. Fortunately, this is not the case here at this convention center. Ornamental pear trees with Indian hawthorn beneath formulate the base of this landscape.

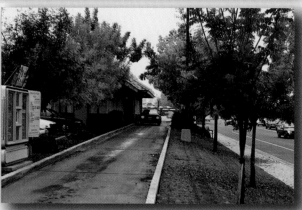

This fast food restaurant drive through is lined with allergy-free Chinese pistache trees. Customers waiting for their food won't be exposed to allergy producing trees on these premises. Imagine what would happen if these trees were olive, mulberry or other allergy producing trees.

This residence is an excellent example of an allergy-free landscape. Plants in this yard include photinia, azaleas, sagos, queen palms, and crape myrtle trees (in the background). Notice the queen palms do not have any flower spikes.

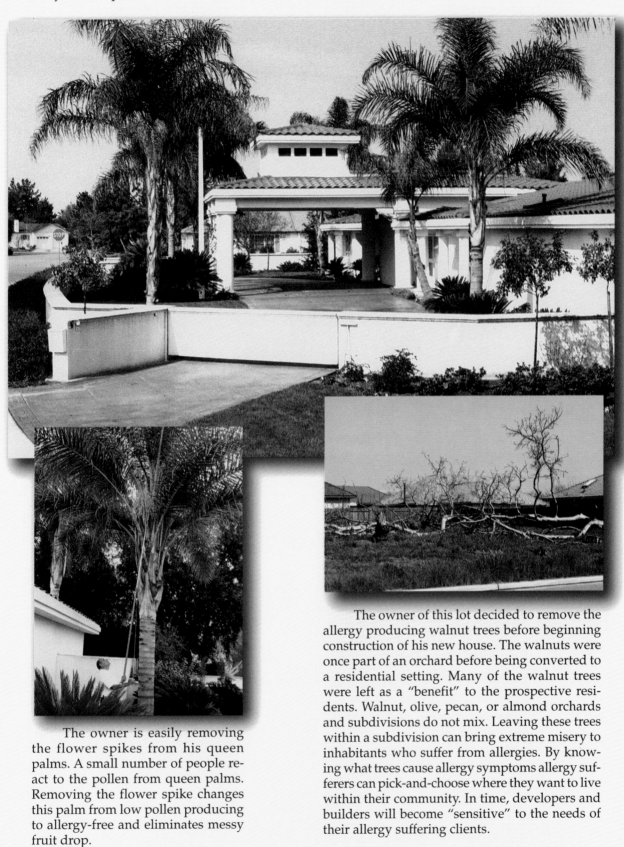

The owner is easily removing the flower spikes from his queen palms. A small number of people react to the pollen from queen palms. Removing the flower spike changes this palm from low pollen producing to allergy-free and eliminates messy fruit drop.

The owner of this lot decided to remove the allergy producing walnut trees before beginning construction of his new house. The walnuts were once part of an orchard before being converted to a residential setting. Many of the walnut trees were left as a "benefit" to the prospective residents. Walnut, olive, pecan, or almond orchards and subdivisions do not mix. Leaving these trees within a subdivision can bring extreme misery to inhabitants who suffer from allergies. By knowing what trees cause allergy symptoms allergy sufferers can pick-and-choose where they want to live within their community. In time, developers and builders will become "sensitive" to the needs of their allergy suffering clients.

Children are hard hit by allergies. Can you tell which one of these kids has allergies? The allergy-free tulips will not give you a clue (or symptom). Some flowers can cause allergy symptoms. Planners and planters of open space should be aware of this.

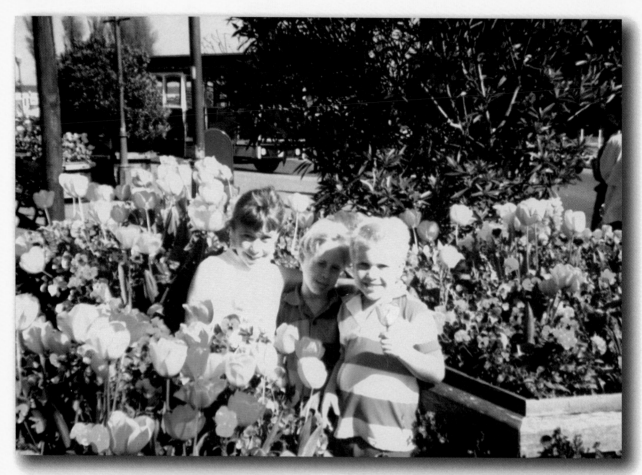

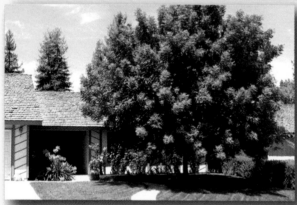

The owners of this residence sprayed their old bermuda grass with a systemic herbicide and replaced it with a fescue lawn. By doing this they have reduced their exposure to pollen from Bermuda grass which is one of the worst allergy producing plants in the United States. Notice the allergy-free Chinese pistache in the front yard.

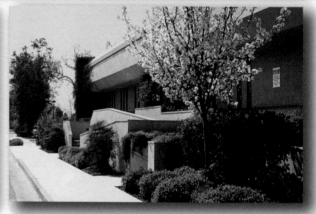

Surrounding this medical building are: evergreen pears, photinias, rhaphiolepis and wheelers' dwarf. All of these plants are allergy-free or low pollen producing. The area around a hospital or doctors office should be an allergy-free zone. Patients entering or leaving such places shouldn't be exposed to potentially harmful allergens especially after an illness or surgery.

Cities and communities need more parks and open space. Architects, landscape contractors and government planners must be aware of allergy producing plants. This young park has sycamore and cedar trees. Interplanting with allergy-free trees and removing the allergy producing trees after four to six years would bring a subtle change to the park. Removing and planting allergy-free plants doesn't have to be done over night. Transitions allow for easy change in our exterior environments.

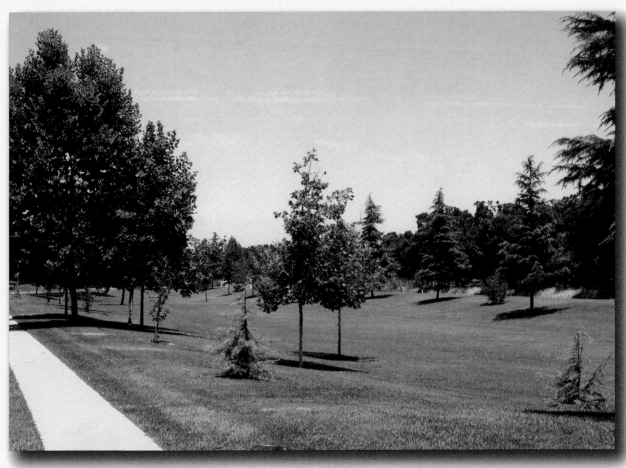

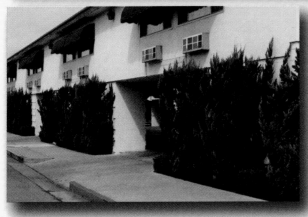

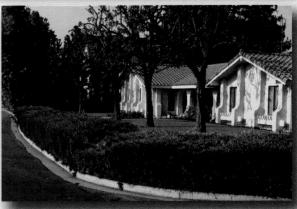

The back of this motel is lined with junipers. Notice the windows and air conditioners above them. If you have allergies and slept with the window open during pollination you could wake up in allergy misery. Businesses will now have the knowledge to provide their customers with on site allergy-free landscapes

This juniper hedge is a good screen and allergy producer. It has out grown its area and looks ratty. Passengers unloading from a vehicle will no doubt brush against the hedge. This type of contact is enough to start allergy symptoms. There are alternative allergy-free shrubs that look better and provide the same or better function.

Shade trees for shopping center parking lots are a great idea. However, using allergy producing sycamores is not. In addition to pollen, sycamores produce a leaf fuzz which is extremely irritating if inhaled or contacts the skin. There are better choices. The tulip tree (*Liroidendron tulipifera*) looks almost identical to the sycamore, yet is allergy-free.

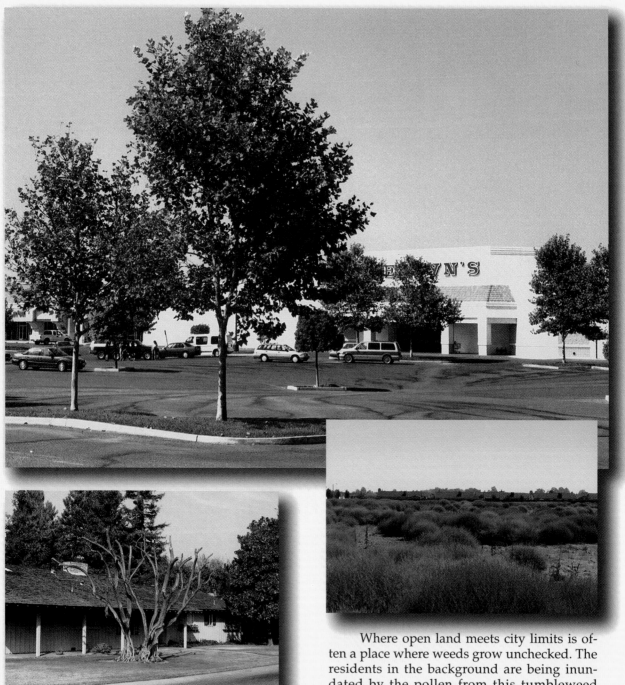

All that remains of this olive tree is the main branches. At this point the tree has lost its aesthetics and should be removed. Planting an allergy-free tree in its place would be the best remedy. Olive trees are messy, high maintenance, and highly allergenic. They should not be used in landscape situations.

Where open land meets city limits is often a place where weeds grow unchecked. The residents in the background are being inundated by the pollen from this tumbleweed colony. Early weed control by plowing this field would have reduced the tumbleweed population to almost zero. There are ordinances against this type of weed growth for fire protection. Why can't we go one step further and protect ourselves from allergy producing weeds by voluntarily killing (plowing) weeds before they pollinate. Everyone will benefit.

The tree on the right is an allergy producing sycamore. The two trees on the left are allergy-free tulips (*Liriodendron tulipifera*). Sycamores can also become brown and dead looking in some areas of the country. Which would you like to have where your live, work or shop?

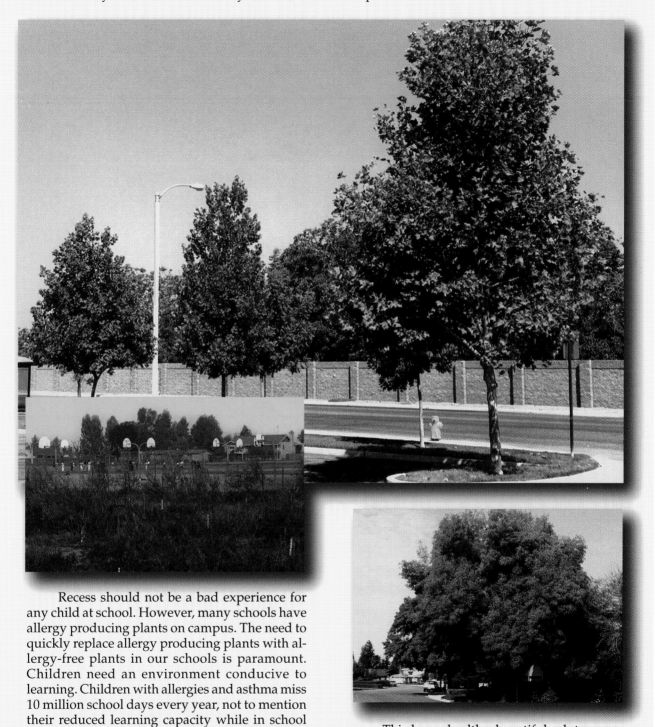

Recess should not be a bad experience for any child at school. However, many schools have allergy producing plants on campus. The need to quickly replace allergy producing plants with allergy-free plants in our schools is paramount. Children need an environment conducive to learning. Children with allergies and asthma miss 10 million school days every year, not to mention their reduced learning capacity while in school and suffering from allergy symptoms. This school received pressure from parents of allergic children to remove these olive trees that were planted on campus. Because of this and other reasons the trees were removed. Allergy producing plants have no business on school grounds. Our tax dollars should not be used in public situations that would cause anyone to become sick or ill.

This large, healthy, beautiful ash tree provides a lot of functional and aesthetic value to the property. Evaluating it strictly on its allergy producing faults may not be a reason for removing it. Proper pruning may be the only thing this tree needs.

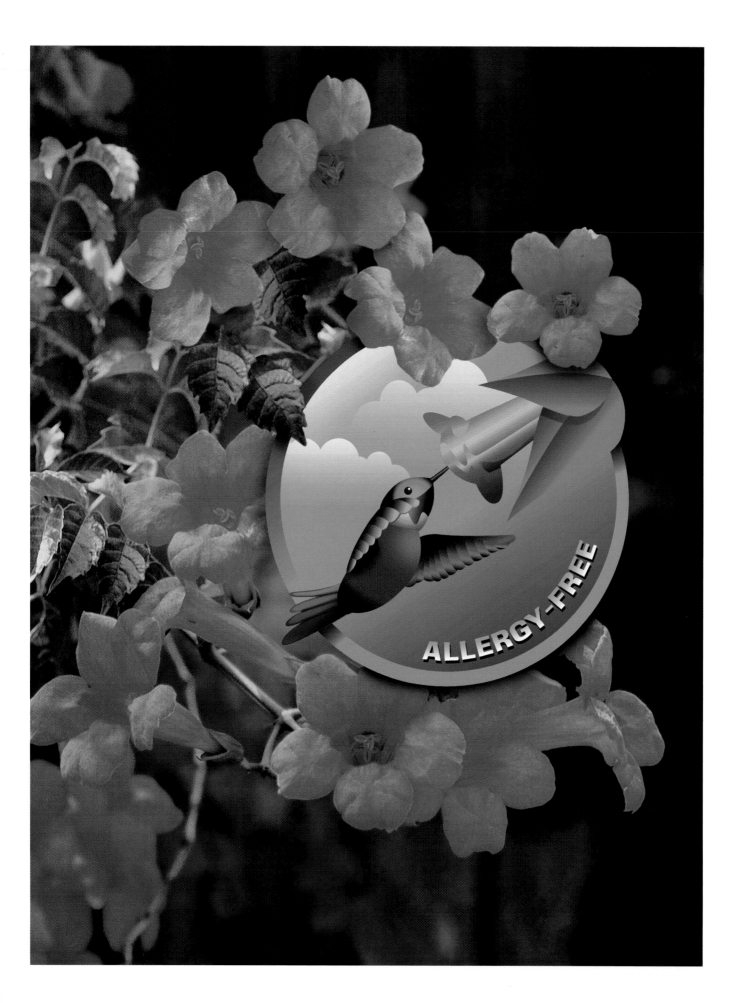

Chapter 8

Replacing Allergy Producing with Allergy-Free Plants

◼ Substituting Plants

This chapter is designed to assist people who would like to remove allergy producing plants from their landscape and replace them with allergy-free plants that have similar characteristics. This chapter will help those who are not plant knowledgeable, or plant lovers who need a quick reference. Either way these charts will get you started.

The charts are designed to give you several choices of allergy-free plants for every allergy producing plant listed. The allergy producing plant is listed at the top of every chart in bold and the **Botanical Name** in italics. In the chart are the allergy-free plants that have similar characteristics including **USDA Zones, Height/Width, Deciduous/Evergreen, Flowers, Fruit/Seed, Messy, Leaf, Water Requirements, Root System** and **Growth Rate.**

The dot(s) indicates the similar characteristics between the allergy producing plant and each allergy-free plant.

One dot means a slight resemblance or similarity of that characteristic between the two plants. Two dots means a moderate similarity, and three dots

a very close similarity.

For example; Acacia - *Acacia spp.* is an allergy producing plant. Jacaranda, podocarpus and silk are allergy-free trees that have some similar characteristics with the acacia tree. The jacaranda tree has only a few similar USDA zones in common and the root systems are only slightly similar to the acacia tree. The Height/Width, Deciduous/Evergreen, Flowers, Leaf, Water Requirements and Growth Rate of the jacaranda and silk tree are all moderately similar to those of the acacia tree. However, in these same categories, the podocarpus has either slightly similar or no similarities or characteristics. The jacaranda and silk tree are both as messy as the acacia tree. The podocarpus is not as messy.

The following charts will indicate the similar attributes of the plants listed as possible substitutions. Study them carefully and try to consider all of the characteristics before making a decision. Use this section as a guide to help you narrow your choices. After selecting several choices look them up in the allergy-free plant chapter for more detailed information. After doing this you should be able to make an intelligent replacement decision.

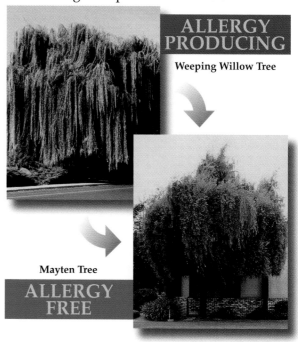

ALLERGY PRODUCING — Ash Tree
Raywood Ash Tree — ALLERGY FREE

ALLERGY PRODUCING — Weeping Willow Tree
Mayten Tree — ALLERGY FREE

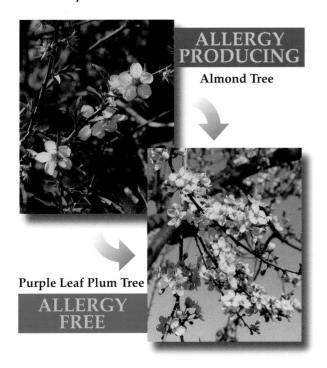

ALLERGY PRODUCING

Almond Tree

Purple Leaf Plum Tree

ALLERGY FREE

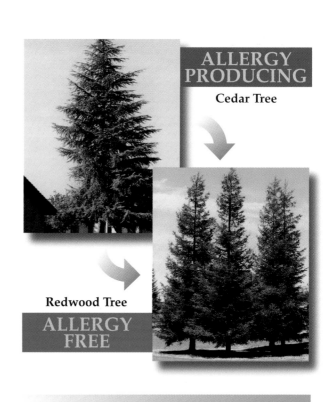

ALLERGY PRODUCING

Cedar Tree

Redwood Tree

ALLERGY FREE

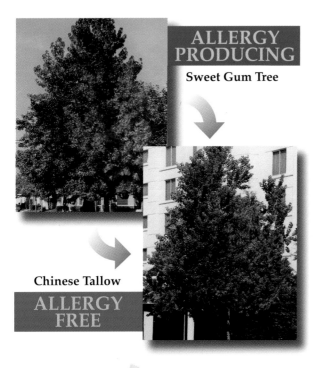

ALLERGY PRODUCING

Sweet Gum Tree

Chinese Tallow

ALLERGY FREE

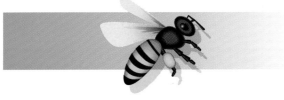

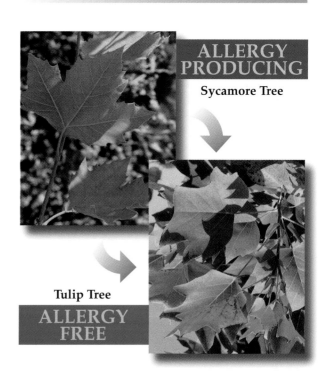

ALLERGY PRODUCING

Sycamore Tree

Tulip Tree

ALLERGY FREE

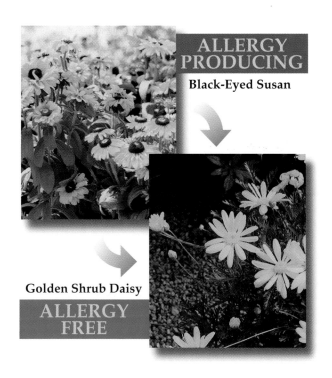

ALLERGY
PRODUCING

Black-Eyed Susan

Golden Shrub Daisy

ALLERGY
FREE

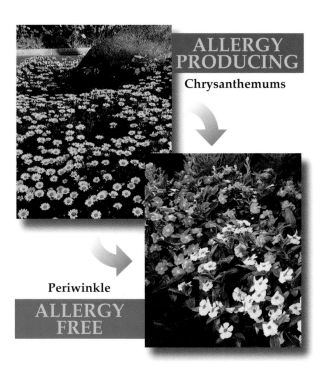

ALLERGY
PRODUCING

Chrysanthemums

Periwinkle

ALLERGY
FREE

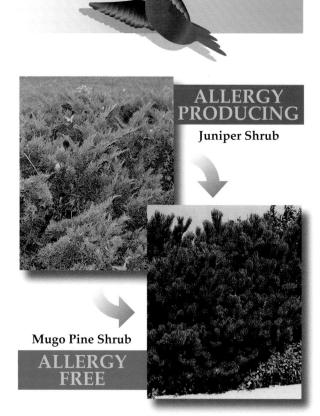

ALLERGY
PRODUCING

Juniper Shrub

Mugo Pine Shrub

ALLERGY
FREE

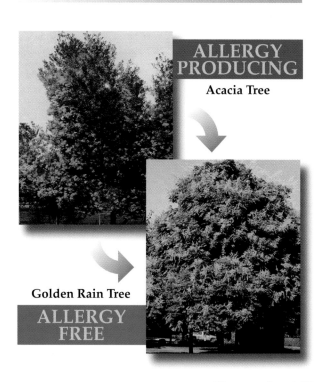

ALLERGY
PRODUCING

Acacia Tree

Golden Rain Tree

ALLERGY
FREE

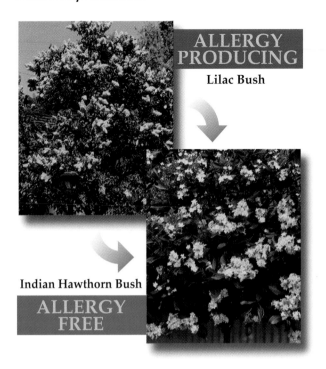

ALLERGY PRODUCING

Lilac Bush

Indian Hawthorn Bush

ALLERGY FREE

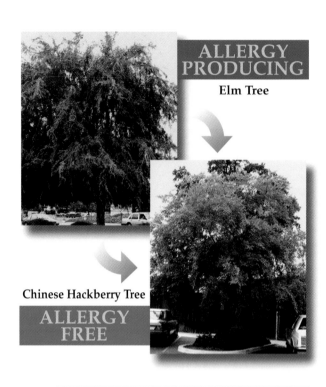

ALLERGY PRODUCING

Elm Tree

Chinese Hackberry Tree

ALLERGY FREE

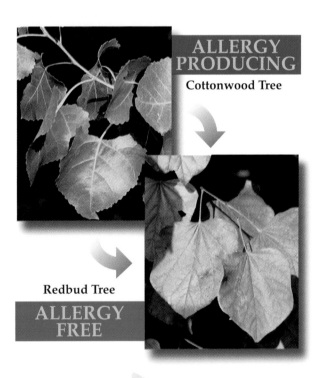

ALLERGY PRODUCING

Cottonwood Tree

Redbud Tree

ALLERGY FREE

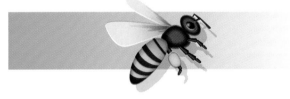

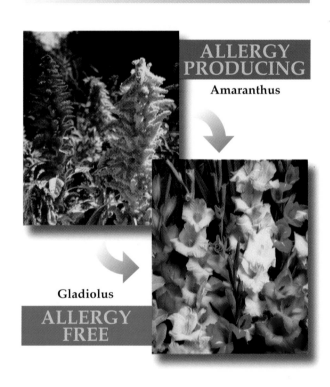

ALLERGY PRODUCING

Amaranthus

Gladiolus

ALLERGY FREE

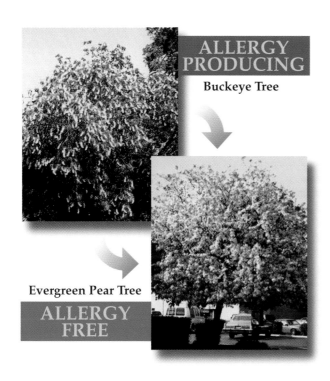

ALLERGY PRODUCING
Buckeye Tree

Evergreen Pear Tree
ALLERGY FREE

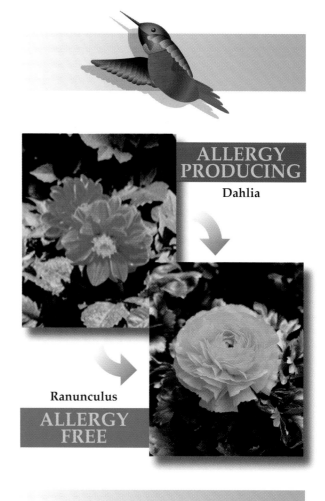

ALLERGY PRODUCING
Dahlia

Ranunculus
ALLERGY FREE

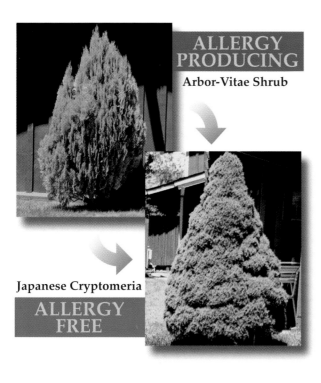

ALLERGY PRODUCING
Arbor-Vitae Shrub

Japanese Cryptomeria
ALLERGY FREE

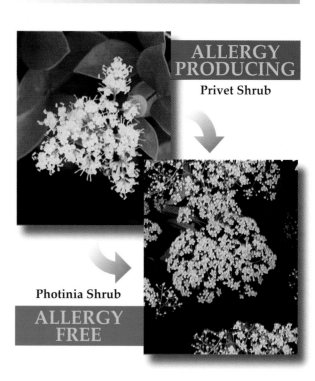

ALLERGY PRODUCING
Privet Shrub

Photinia Shrub
ALLERGY FREE

• Slightly Similar •• Moderately Similar ••• Very Similar

Trees

Allergy Producing Tree:
ACACIA - *Acacia spp.*

Allergy Free Replacement Trees:

	USDA ZONES	HEIGHT/WIDTH	DECID./EVERGREEN	FLOWERS	FRUIT/SEED	MESSY	LEAF	WATER REQ.	ROOT SYSTEM	GROWTH RATE
Jacaranda - *Jacaranda acutifolia*	•	••	••	••	••	•••	••	••	•	••
Golden Rain Tree - *Koelrueteria paniculata*	••	••	••	••		•		••	•	
Silk Tree - *Albizia julibrissin*	•	••	••	••	••	•••	••	••	•	••

Allergy Producing Tree:
ALDER - *Alnus spp.*

Allergy Free Replacement Trees:

	USDA ZONES	HEIGHT/WIDTH	DECID./EVERGREEN	FLOWERS	FRUIT/SEED	MESSY	LEAF	WATER REQ.	ROOT SYSTEM	GROWTH RATE
Carolina Cherry - *Prunus caroliniana*	•	•				•				••
Tulip Tree - *Liriodendron tulipifera*	••	•	•••					•		••
Redwood - *Sequoia sempervirens*	••	•						•		••
Canary Island Pine - *Pinus canariensis*	••	•						•		••
Ornamental Pear - *Pyrus calleryana*	••		••				•	•		•

Allergy Producing Tree:
ALMOND - *Prunus dulcis*

Allergy Free Replacement Trees:

	USDA ZONES	HEIGHT/WIDTH	DECID./EVERGREEN	FLOWERS	FRUIT/SEED	MESSY	LEAF	WATER REQ.	ROOT SYSTEM	GROWTH RATE
Dogwood - *Cornus florida*	•	•	•••	•			•			
Chinese Hackberry - *Celtis sinensis*	•		•••				•	•		•
Purple Leaf Plum - *Prunus cerasifera 'Atropurpurea'*	•	•••	•••	••	••	•	•	•	••	••
California Bay Laurel - *Umbellularia californica*	•	•		•			•	•	•	

Allergy Producing Tree:
ASH - *Fraxinus spp.*

Allergy Free Replacement Trees:

	USDA ZONES	HEIGHT/WIDTH	DECID./EVERGREEN	FLOWERS	FRUIT/SEED	MESSY	LEAF	WATER REQ.	ROOT SYSTEM	GROWTH RATE
Raywood Ash* - *Fraxinus oxycarpa 'Raywood'*	•••	•••	••	••			••	•••	•••	•••
Podocarpus - *Podocarpus gracilior*	•	•						•		
Golden Rain Tree - *Koelreuteria paniculata*	••	••	•••		•	•		•		
Chinese Pistache - *Pistacia chinensis*	•	••	•••		•			•		
Chinese Hackberry - *Celtis sinensis*	•	••	•••							

*Note: Raywood ash trees are hybrids and do not produce flowers or pollen.

• Slightly Similar   •• Moderately Similar   ••• Very Similar

Trees

Allergy Producing Tree:
BIRCH - *Betula spp.*
Allergy Free Replacement Trees:

	USDA ZONES	HEIGHT/WIDTH	DECID./EVERGREEN	FLOWERS	FRUIT/SEED	MESSY	LEAF	WATER REQ.	ROOT SYSTEM	GROWTH RATE
Redbud - *Cercis occidentalis*	••	•	•••		•					
Podocarpus - *Podocarpus gracilior*	••	•								
Maytens - *Matenus boria*	••	•								
Weeping Fig - *Ficus benjamina*	•	•						•	•	

Allergy Producing Tree:
BUCKEYE - *Aesculus californica*
Allergy Free Replacement Trees:

	USDA ZONES	HEIGHT/WIDTH	DECID./EVERGREEN	FLOWERS	FRUIT/SEED	MESSY	LEAF	WATER REQ.	ROOT SYSTEM	GROWTH RATE
Evergreen Pear - *Pyrus Kawakamii*	••	••	••	•	•	•	•		•	
Golden Rain Tree - *Koelreuteria paniculata*	••	••	••	•	•	•		•	•	•
Silk Tree - *Albizia julibrissin*	••	••	••	•	•	•				
Western Catalpa - *Catalpa speciosa*	••		•			•			•	

Allergy Producing Tree:
CEDAR - *Cedrus spp.*
Allergy Free Replacement Trees:

	USDA ZONES	HEIGHT/WIDTH	DECID./EVERGREEN	FLOWERS	FRUIT/SEED	MESSY	LEAF	WATER REQ.	ROOT SYSTEM	GROWTH RATE
Canary Island Pine - *Pinus canariensis*	••	••	•••		•		•	•	•	•
Redwood - *Sequoia sempervirens*	••	••	•••				•			•
White Fir - *Abies concolor*	••	•	•••		•				•	

Allergy Producing Tree:
CHESTNUT - *Castanea spp.*
Allergy Free Replacement Trees:

	USDA ZONES	HEIGHT/WIDTH	DECID./EVERGREEN	FLOWERS	FRUIT/SEED	MESSY	LEAF	WATER REQ.	ROOT SYSTEM	GROWTH RATE
Carolina Cherry - *Prunus caroliniana*	••	•		•			••		•	
Southern Magnolia - *Magnolia grandiflora*	••	••		•	•	•	•	••	•	•
Golden Rain Tree - *Koelreuteria paniculata*	••	•	•••	•	•	•		•	•	•
Chinese Tallow - *Sapium sebiferum*	•	•	•••		•					

Allergy Producing Tree:
COTTONWOOD - *Populus spp.*
Allergy Free Replacement Trees:

	USDA ZONES	HEIGHT/WIDTH	DECID./EVERGREEN	FLOWERS	FRUIT/SEED	MESSY	LEAF	WATER REQ.	ROOT SYSTEM	GROWTH RATE
Redbud - *Cercis occidentalis*	•••		•••				•			
Tulip Tree - *Liriodenron tulipifera*	••	•	•••					•		••
Orchid Tree - *Bauhinia vareigata*	•		•••					••		•
Redwood - *Sequoia sempervirens*	•	••						•		•

• Slightly Similar	•• Moderately Similar	••• Very Similar

Trees

Allergy Producing Tree: ELM - *Ulmus spp.*
Allergy Free Replacement Trees:

	USDA ZONES	HEIGHT/WIDTH	DECID./EVERGREEN	FLOWERS	FRUIT/SEED	MESSY	LEAF	WATER REQ.	ROOT SYSTEM	GROWTH RATE
Chinese Hackberry - *Celtis sinensis*	•	••	•••			•	•••	••		••
Evergreen Pear - *Pyrus kawakamii*	•	••	•••		•	•		••	•	•••
Chinese Tallow - *Sapium sebiferum*	•	••	•••		•		•	••	••	•••

Allergy Producing Tree: EUCALYPTUS - *Eucalyptus spp.*
Allergy Free Replacement Trees:

	USDA ZONES	HEIGHT/WIDTH	DECID./EVERGREEN	FLOWERS	FRUIT/SEED	MESSY	LEAF	WATER REQ.	ROOT SYSTEM	GROWTH RATE
Ash Eucalyptus - *Eucalyptus cinerea*	••	•	••	••	•	••	••	••	••	••
Red Iron Bark Eucalyptus - *Eucalyptus sideroxylon*	••	•	••	••	•	••	••	••	••	••
Southern Magnolia - *Magnolia grandiflora*	•	••	•••	•	•	•			•	

Allergy Producing Tree: MAPLE - *Acer spp.*
Allergy Free Replacement Trees:

	USDA ZONES	HEIGHT/WIDTH	DECID./EVERGREEN	FLOWERS	FRUIT/SEED	MESSY	LEAF	WATER REQ.	ROOT SYSTEM	GROWTH RATE
Golden Rain Tree - *Koelreuteria paniculata*	••	•	••		•			•		•
Tulip Tree - *Liroidendron tulipifera*	••	•	••					•		•
Saucer Magnolia - *Magnolia soulangiana*	••	•	••					•		••
Chinese Tallow - *Sapium sebiferum*	•	•	••		•			•	•	•

Allergy Producing Tree: MESQUITE - *Prosopis spp.*
Allergy Free Replacement Trees:

	USDA ZONES	HEIGHT/WIDTH	DECID./EVERGREEN	FLOWERS	FRUIT/SEED	MESSY	LEAF	WATER REQ.	ROOT SYSTEM	GROWTH RATE
Silk Tree - *Albizia julibrissin*	••	•	••	••	••	••	••			•
Jacaranda - *Jacaranda acutifolia*	••	•	••	••	••	••	••			•
Podocarpus - *Podocarpus gracilior*	••	•					•			•

Allergy Producing Tree: MULBERRY - *Morus spp.*
Allergy Free Replacement Trees:

	USDA ZONES	HEIGHT/WIDTH	DECID./EVERGREEN	FLOWERS	FRUIT/SEED	MESSY	LEAF	WATER REQ.	ROOT SYSTEM	GROWTH RATE
Chinese Tallow - *Sapium sebiferum*	•	••	•••					•	•••	••
Western Catalpa - *Catalpa speciosa*	•••	••	•••				•	•		•
Raywood Ash - *Fraxinus oxycarpa 'Raywood'*	••	••	•••		•			•	•••	•••
Evergreen Pear - *Pyrus kawakamii*	•	•	••							•
Camphor Tree - *Cinnamomum camphora*	•	•								•

• Slightly Similar   •• Moderately Similar   ••• Very Similar

Trees

Allergy Producing Tree: OLIVE - *Olea europaea*
Allergy Free Replacement Trees:

	USDA ZONES	HEIGHT/WIDTH	DECID./EVERGREEN	FLOWERS	FRUIT/SEED	MESSY	LEAF	WATER REQ.	ROOT SYSTEM	GROWTH RATE
Purple Leaf Plum - *Prunus cerasifera 'Atropurpurea'*	••	••		•	••	•		•	•	
Crape Myrtle - *Lagerstroemia indica*	••	••		•			•	•	•	••
Chinese Pistache - *Pistacia chinensis*	••	•			•			•	•	••
Silk Tree - *Albizia julibrissin*	•••	••		•	••	•		•		
Camphor - *Cinnamomum camphora*	•••	••	•••		•			•		•
Podocarpus - *Podocarpus gracilior*	•••	•	•••				•	•	•	•••
Maytens Tree - *Maytenus boria*	••	••	•••				••	•	•	••

Allergy Producing Tree: PECAN - *Carya Illinoensis*
Allergy Free Replacement Trees:

	USDA ZONES	HEIGHT/WIDTH	DECID./EVERGREEN	FLOWERS	FRUIT/SEED	MESSY	LEAF	WATER REQ.	ROOT SYSTEM	GROWTH RATE
Tulip Tree - *Liriodendron tulipifera*	••	•••	••					•	•	•
Western Catalpa - *Catalpa speciosa*	••	•••	•		•	•		•	•	•
Southern Magnolia - *Magnolia grandiflora*	••		•••		•	•	•	••		
Redwood - *Sequoia sempervirens*	••		••							•

Allergy Producing Tree: CALIFORNIA PEPPER - *Schinus molle*
Allergy Free Replacement Trees:

	USDA ZONES	HEIGHT/WIDTH	DECID./EVERGREEN	FLOWERS	FRUIT/SEED	MESSY	LEAF	WATER REQ.	ROOT SYSTEM	GROWTH RATE
Silk Tree - *Albizia julibrissin*	••		•		•	••		•		••
Jacaranda - *Jacaranda acutifolia*	•		•		•	••		•		••
Podocarpus - *Podocarpus gracilior*	•••	•••	•				•	•		
Maytens Tree - *Maytenus boria*	••	•••					•		•	

Allergy Producing Tree: PRIVET - *Ligustrum spp.*
Allergy Free Replacement Trees:

	USDA ZONES	HEIGHT/WIDTH	DECID./EVERGREEN	FLOWERS	FRUIT/SEED	MESSY	LEAF	WATER REQ.	ROOT SYSTEM	GROWTH RATE
Carolina Cherry - *Prunus caroliniana*	••	•	•••	••	•	•	•	•	•	•
Xylosma - *Xylosma congestum*	••	•••	••	•			•	••	••	••
California Bay Laurel - *Umbellularia californica*	••	•	•••	•				••	•	
Escallonia - *Escallonia spp.*	••	••	••	••		•		••		••
Photinia - *Photinia fraseri*	••	••	•••	•••	•			••	••	••

• Slightly Similar   •• Moderately Similar   ••• Very Similar

Trees

Allergy Producing Tree:
SWEET GUM - *Liquidambar styraciflua*

Allergy Free Replacement Trees:

	USDA ZONES	HEIGHT/WIDTH	DECID/EVERGREEN	FLOWERS	FRUIT/SEED	MESSY	LEAF	WATER REQ.	ROOT SYSTEM	GROWTH RATE
Ginkgo - *Ginkgo biloba*	••	•••	••		•		•	•		
Southern Magnolia - *Magnolia grandiflora*	••	••			•	••				
Tulip Tree - *Liriodendron tulipifera*	••	••	•••				•••	••		•••
Raywood Ash - *Fraxinus oxycarpa 'Raywood'*	••		•••				•	••	•••	•••
Chinese Tallow - *Sapium sebiferum*	•••	••	•••		•	•		••	•••	••

Allergy Producing Tree:
SYCAMORE - *Platanus spp.*

Allergy Free Replacement Trees:

	USDA ZONES	HEIGHT/WIDTH	DECID/EVERGREEN	FLOWERS	FRUIT/SEED	MESSY	LEAF	WATER REQ.	ROOT SYSTEM	GROWTH RATE
Tulip Tree - *Liriodendron tulipifera*	••	••	•••				•••	••	•	•••
Western Catapla - *Catalpa speciosa*	•••	••	•••		•	••	•	•		••
Argyle Apple - *Eucalyptus cinerea*	••	••					•	••	••	•••

Allergy Producing Tree:
TAMARISK - *Tamarix spp.*

Allergy Free Replacement Trees:

	USDA ZONES	HEIGHT/WIDTH	DECID/EVERGREEN	FLOWERS	FRUIT/SEED	MESSY	LEAF	WATER REQ.	ROOT SYSTEM	GROWTH RATE
Podocarpus - *Podocarpus macrphyllus*	•••	••	•				••	•		
Fountain Butterfly - *Buddleia alternifolia*	•	••	•	••		•				••
Argyle Apple - *Eucalyptus cinerea*	•	•	•••					•		•••
Raywood Ash - *Fraxinus oxycarpa 'Raywood'*	••	•						•		•••
Xylosma - *Xylosma congestum*	•	•	•••	••				•		••

Allergy Producing Tree:
TREE-OF-HEAVEN - *Ailanthus altissima*

Allergy Free Replacement Trees:

	USDA ZONES	HEIGHT/WIDTH	DECID/EVERGREEN	FLOWERS	FRUIT/SEED	MESSY	LEAF	WATER REQ.	ROOT SYSTEM	GROWTH RATE
Canary Island Pine - *Pinus canariensis*	••	••								••
Golden Rain Tree - *Koelreuteria paniculata*	••	•	•••	•						
Southern Magnolia - *Magnolia grandiflora*	••	••		•		•				

Allergy Producing Tree:
WALNUT - Juglans spp.

Allergy Free Replacement Trees:

	USDA ZONES	HEIGHT/WIDTH	DECID/EVERGREEN	FLOWERS	FRUIT/SEED	MESSY	LEAF	WATER REQ.	ROOT SYSTEM	GROWTH RATE
Chinese Pistache - *Pistacia chinensis*	••	••	•••		•			•	•	
Silk Tree - *Albizia julibrissin*	••	••	•••		•	•		••	•	••
Jacaranda - *Jacaranda acutifolia*	•	••	•••		•	•		•		••

• Slightly Similar	•• Moderately Similar	••• Very Similar

Trees

Allergy Producing Tree:
WALNUT - *Juglans spp.* (CON'T)
Allergy Free Replacement Trees:

	USDA ZONES	HEIGHT/WIDTH	DECID./EVERGREEN	FLOWERS	FRUIT/SEED	MESSY	LEAF	WATER REQ.	ROOT SYSTEM	GROWTH RATE
Chinese Hackberry - *Celtis sinensis*	•	••	•••					•		•
Loquat - *Eriobotrya japonica*	••	•		•	••		••	•	•	•••
Chinese Tallow - *Sapium sebiferum*	•	••	•••			•	•	••		•••
Golden Rain Tree - *Koelreuteria paniculata*	••	•	•••					•		

Allergy Producing Tree:
WILLOW - *Salix spp.*
Allergy Free Replacement Trees:

	USDA ZONES	HEIGHT/WIDTH	DECID./EVERGREEN	FLOWERS	FRUIT/SEED	MESSY	LEAF	WATER REQ.	ROOT SYSTEM	GROWTH RATE
Camphor Tree - *Cinnamomum camphora*	•	••						•		
Maytens Tree - *Maytenus boria*	•						•			
Argyle Apple - *Eucalyptus cinerea*	••	•				•	•	•		•••
Chinese Tallow - *Sapium sebiferum*	•	••	•••					••	••	••
Australian Tea Tree - *Leptospermum laevigatum*	•							•		

Shrubs

Allergy Producing Shrub:
CEANOTHUS - *Ceanothus spp.*
Allergy Free Replacement Shrubs:

	USDA ZONES	SIZE	FLOWERS	LEAF	WATER REQ.	GROWTH RATE
Escallonia - *Escallonia spp.*	••	••	••	••		
Indian Hawthorn - *Rhaphiolepis indica*	••	••	•			
Manzanita - *Arctostaphylos hookerii*	••	••	•		•••	•
Coyote Brush - *Baccharis pilularis*	••	•		•	•••	•
English Holly - *Ilex aquifolium*	••	•	••			

Allergy Producing Shrub:
ELDERBERRY - *Sambucus spp.*
Allergy Free Replacement Shrubs:

	USDA ZONES	SIZE	FLOWERS	LEAF	WATER REQ.	GROWTH RATE
Spiraea - *Spiraea bumalda 'Anthony Waterer'*	••		•		•	
David Viburnum - *Viburnum davidii*	••	••	••	•	••	•
Pineapple Guava - *Feijoa sellowiana*	••	•	•		••	•
English Holly - *Ilex aquifolium*	••	•				
Forsythia - *Forsythia intermedia*	••	••	•	•	•	•

| • Slightly Similar | •• Moderately Similar | ••• Very Similar |

Shrubs

Allergy Producing Shrub:
FOUNTAIN GRASS - *Pennisetum setaceum*

Allergy Free Replacement Shrubs:

	USDA ZONES	SIZE	FLOWERS	LEAF	WATER REQ.	GROWTH RATE
New Zealand Flax - *Phormuim tenax*	••	•		•		
Glossy Abelia - *Abelia grandiflora*	••	•				
Breath of Heaven - *Diosma (Coleonema) ericoides*	••	•••	•		•••	•

Allergy Producing Shrub:
JUNIPER - *Juniperus spp.*

Allergy Free Replacement Shrubs:

	USDA ZONES	SIZE	FLOWERS	LEAF	WATER REQ.	GROWTH RATE
Mugo Pine - *Pinus mugo mugo*	••	••		•	•	
Lantana - *Lantana camera*	••	••			••	••
Golden Shrub Daisy - *Euryops pectinatus*	•	••				
Hooker Manzanita - *Arctostaphylos hookeri*	••	••			••	••
Creeping Manzanita - *Arctostaphylos uva-ursi*	••	••			••	••
Bearberry Cotoneaster - *Cotoneaster dammeri*	•••	••			•	

Allergy Producing Shrub:
LILAC - *Syringa spp.*

Allergy Free Replacement Shrubs:

	USDA ZONES	SIZE	FLOWERS	LEAF	WATER REQ.	GROWTH RATE
Camellia - *Camellia japonica*	•	••	••	•••	••	••
Indian Hawthorn - *Rhaphiolepis indica*	•	•	••	•	••	••
Dwarf Spiraea - *Spiraea bumalda 'Anthony Waterer'*	•••	•	••		••	••
Common Snowball - *Viburnum opulus 'Roseum'*	••	••	••	•	••	

Allergy Producing Shrub:
COFFEEBERRY - *Rhamnus spp.*

Allergy Free Replacement Shrubs:

	USDA ZONES	SIZE	FLOWERS	LEAF	WATER REQ.	GROWTH RATE
Indian Hawthorn - *Rhaphiolepis indica*	••			•••		•
Coyote Brush - *Baccharis pilularis*	••	••			••	••
Common Lantana - *Lantana camera*	••	•			••	••

Allergy Producing Shrub:
PAMPUS GRASS - *Cortaderia selloana*

Allergy Free Replacement Shrubs:

	USDA ZONES	SIZE	FLOWERS	LEAF	WATER REQ.	GROWTH RATE
Sago - *Cycas revoluta*	••	•			••	
Glossy Abelia - *Abelia grandiflora*	•••	••			••	•
New Zealand Flax - *Phormium tenax*	•••	•••		••	••	•••
Matilija Poppy - *Romneya coulteri*	••	•••			••	••

Turf Grass

The following chart provides information about the replacement grasses. It is not a comparison chart like the previous tree and shrub charts. Moreover, it categorizes the grasses into their respective preferred growing seasons and their invasive characteristics. A cool season grass grows best from the fall through spring. They grow well in the summer months but need consistent irrigation and can have fungal problems in times of hot, humid summers. Cool season grasses generally stay green all year long (except annual ryegrass). Warm season grasses grow best in the spring through end of summer or beginning of fall. Warm season grasses usually go dormate in areas of moderate to cold winters. Remember, the grasses listed below are all allergy producing if they are not mowed regularly. Our main focus is to replace bermuda grass with a less allergy provoking grass.

Allergy Producing Grass:
BERMUDA - *Cynodon dactylon*
Allergy Free Replacement Grasses:

	COOL SEASON	WARM SEASON	EVERGREEN	DECIDUOUS	INVASIVE
Fescue - *Festuca rubra*	•••		•••		
Kentucky Bluegrass - *Poa pratensis*	•••		•••		
Hybrid Bermuda - *Cynodon spp.*		•••		•••	•••

Flowers

There are several genera of flowers that can cause allergy symptoms. The following chart provides information about the replacement flowers. It is not a comparison chart like the previous tree and shrub charts. Moreover, it categorizes the allergy-free flowers into their respective characteristics. Refer to the flower section in the allergy-free chapter for more detailed information. The allergy producing flower is listed in bold capitol letters with the Botanical Name in italics. Under flower season "Sp" is Spring, "S" is Summer, "F" is Fall and "W" is Winter.

Allergy Producing Flower:
AMARANTHUS - *Amaranthus spp.*
Allergy Free Replacement Flowers:

	USDA ZONES	FLOWER SEASON	HEIGHT	WHITE	RED/PINK	BLUE/PURPLE	YELLOW/ORANGE	MULTI-COLOR
Hollyhock - *Alcea rosea*	ALL	S	5' - 9'	•	•	•	•	
Columbine - *Aquilegia spp.*	ALL	S	4'	•	•	•	•	
Gladiolus - *Gladiolus spp.*	ALL	Sp/S	2' - 6'	•	•	•	•	•

Allergy Producing Flower:
BLACK-EYED SUSAN - *Rudbeckia hirta*
Allergy Free Replacement Flowers:

	USDA ZONES	FLOWER SEASON	HEIGHT	WHITE	RED/PINK	BLUE/PURPLE	YELLOW/ORANGE	MULTI-COLOR
Periwinkle - *Catharanthus roseus (Vinca rosea)*	ALL	S/F	1' - 3'	•	•	•		•
Carnation - *Dianthus spp.*	ALL	Sp/S	1-1/2'	•	•		•	
Bougainvillea - *Bougainvillea spp.*	10,11	S	up to15'	•	•	•	•	•

*Note: Bougainvilleas can be grown in many other USDA zones. However, they will need protection from frost. Bougainvilleas are used above as an annual or perennial replacement vine.

Flowers

Allergy Producing Flower:
CHRYSANTHEMUM - *Chrysanthemum spp.*
Allergy Free Replacement Shrubs:

	USDA ZONES	FLOWER SEASON	HEIGHT	WHITE	RED/PINK	BLUE/PURPLE	YELLOW/ORANGE	MULTI-COLOR
Periwinkle - *Catharanthus roseus (Vinca rosea)*	ALL	S/F	1' - 3'	•	•	•		•
Carnation - *Dianthus spp.*	ALL	Sp/S	1-1/2'	•	•		•	
Golden Shrub Daisy - *Euryops pectinatus*	9	Sp/S/F	3' - 6'				•	

Allergy Producing Flower:
DAHLIA - *Dahlia spp.*
Allergy Free Replacement Shrubs:

	USDA ZONES	FLOWER SEASON	HEIGHT	WHITE	RED/PINK	BLUE/PURPLE	YELLOW/ORANGE	MULTI-COLOR
Hollyhock - *Alcea rosea*	ALL	S	5' - 9'	•		•	•	
Gladiolus - *Gadiolus spp.*	ALL	Sp/S/F	2' - 6'	•		•	•	•
Iris - *Iris spp.*	ALL	Sp/S	1' - 7'	•		•	•	•
Ranunculus - *Ranunculus asiaticus*	ALL	Sp/S	2'	•			•	

Allergy Producing Flower:
SUNFLOWER - *Helianthus annuus*
Allergy Free Replacement Shrubs:

	USDA ZONES	FLOWER SEASON	HEIGHT	WHITE	RED/PINK	BLUE/PURPLE	YELLOW/ORANGE	MULTI-COLOR
Hollyhock - *Alcea rosea*	ALL	S	5' - 9'	•	•	•	•	
Canna - *Canna spp.*	ALL	S/F	3' - 6'	•	•	•	•	•

Allergy Producing Flower:
ZINNIA - *Zinnia spp.*
Allergy Free Replacement Shrubs:

	USDA ZONES	FLOWER SEASON	HEIGHT	WHITE	RED/PINK	BLUE/PURPLE	YELLOW/ORANGE	MULTI-COLOR
Begonia - *Begonia spp.*	ALL	Sp/S	6" - 5'	•	•		•	
Periwinkle - *Catharanthus roseus (Vinca rosea)*	ALL	Sp/S/F	1' - 2'	•	•	•		•

*Note: Some USDA zone plants must be used indoors.

illustrations

LEAF SHAPES

 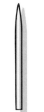 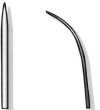 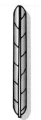 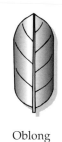 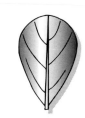 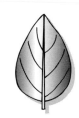 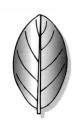

| Subutate | Acicular | Filiform | Linear | Oblong | Ovate | Obovate | Elliptic |

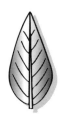 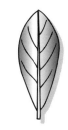 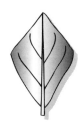 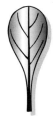 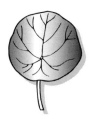 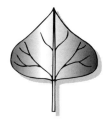 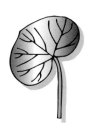

| Lanceolate | Oblanceolate | Rhomboidal | Spatulate | Orbicular | Deltoid | Reniform |

LEAF APICES

| Acute | Acuminate | Aristate | Cuspidate | Mucronate | Obtuse | Retuse | Emarginate |

LEAF BASES

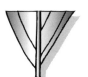 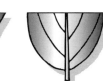   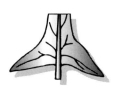

| Cuneate | Attenuate | Obtuse | Cordate | Auriculate | Sagittate | Hastate |

    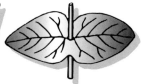

| Truncate | Oblique | Peltate | Perfoliate | Connate-perfoliate | Sheathing | Decurrent |

LEAF TYPES

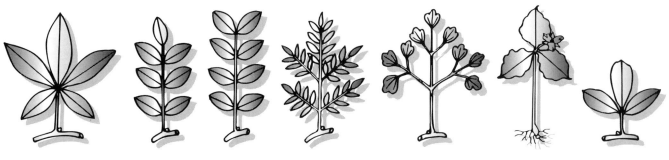

Palmate or Digitate Odd-Pinnate Even-Pinnate Bipinnate Biternate Trifoliate Plant Trifoliate Leaf

FRUITS & NUTS

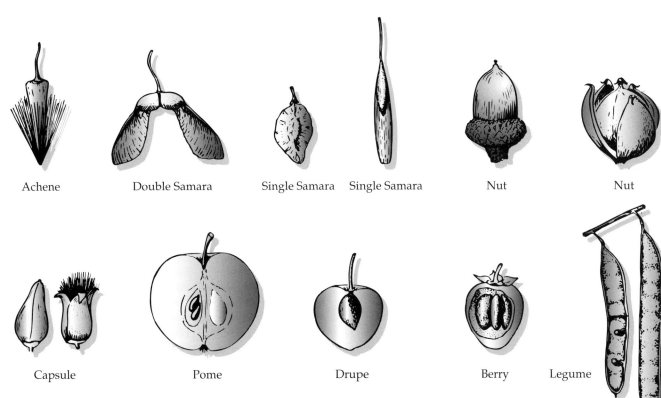

Achene Double Samara Single Samara Single Samara Nut Nut

Capsule Pome Drupe Berry Legume

FLOWER STRUCTURE

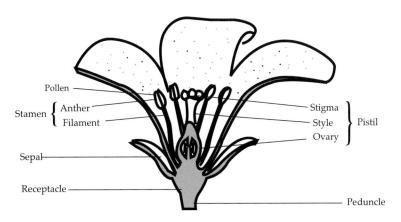

Pollen

Stamen { Anther
         Filament

Stigma
Style
Ovary } Pistil

Sepal

Receptacle

Peduncle

LEAF MARGINS

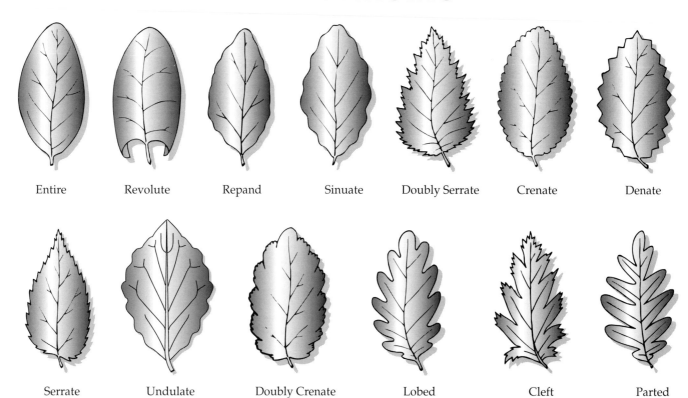

Entire Revolute Repand Sinuate Doubly Serrate Crenate Denate

Serrate Undulate Doubly Crenate Lobed Cleft Parted

FLOWER ARRANGMENTS

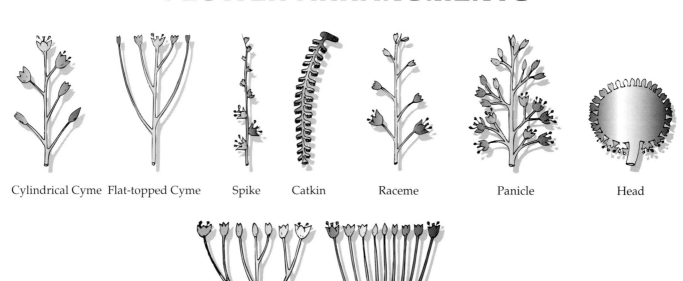

Cylindrical Cyme Flat-topped Cyme Spike Catkin Raceme Panicle Head

Corymb Umbel

official
state trees

– UNITED STATES OFFICIAL STATE TREES –

Year	State	Tree
1949	Alabama	Southern pine *Pinus* spp.
1962	Alaska	Sitka spruce *Picea sitchensis*
1954	Arizona	palo verde *Cercidium* spp.
1939	Arkansas	pine *Pinus* spp.
1972	California	coast redwood *Sequoia sempervirens* and giant sequoia *Sequoiadendron giganteum*
1939	Colorado	blue spruce *Picea pungens*
1947	Connecticut	white oak *Quercus alba*
1939	Delaware	American holly *Ilex opaca*
1960	Dist. of Columbia	scarlet oak *Quercus coccinea*
1953	Flordia	Sabal palm *Sabal palmetto*
1937	Georgia	Live Oak *Quercus virginiana*
1959	Hawaii	candlenut *Aleurites moluccana*
1935	Idaho	western white pine *Pinus monticola*
1908	Illinois	native oak *Quercus* spp.
1931	Indiana	tulip tree *Liriodendron tulipifera*
1961	Iowa	oak *Quercus* spp.
1937	Kansas	cottonwood *Populus* spp.
1956	Kentucky	yellow-poplar *Liriodendron tulipifera*
1963	Louisiana	baldcypress *Taxodium distichum*
1945	Maine	eastern white pine *Pinus strobus*
1941	Maryland	white oak *Quercus alba*
1941	Massachusetts	American elm *Ulmus americana*
1955	Michigan	eastern white pine Pinus strobus
1953	Minnesota	red pine *Pinus resinosa*
1938	Mississippi	magnolia *Magnolia gradiflora*
1955	Missouri	flowering dogwood *Cornus florida*
1949	Montana	ponderosa pine *Pinus ponderosa*
1937	Nebraska	American elm *Ulmus americana*
1953	Nevada	singleleaf pinon *Pinus monophylla*
1947	New Hampshire	white birch *Betula papyrifera*
1950	New Jersey	red oak *Quercus rubra*
1949	New Mexico	pinyon *Pinus edulis*
1956	New York	sugar maple *Acer saccharum*
1963	North Carolina	pine *Pinus* spp.
1947	North Dakota	American elm *Ulmus americana*
1953	Ohio	Ohio buckeye *Aesculus glabra*
1937	Oklahoma	redbud *Cercis canadensis*
1939	Oregon	Douglas-fir *Pseudotsuga menziesii*
1931	Pennsylvania	eastern hemlock *Tsuga canadensis*
1964	Rhode Island	red maple *Acer rubrum*
1939	South Carolina	palmetto *Sabal palmetto*
1947	South Dakota	Black Hills spruce *Picea glauca var. densata*
1947	Tennessee	tulip poplar *Liriodendron tulipifera*
1919	Texas	pecan *Carya illinensis*
1933	Utah	blue spruce *Picea pungens*
1949	Vermont	sugar maple *Acer saccharum*
1956	Virginia	flowering dogwood *Cornus florida*
1947	Washington	western hemlock *Tsuga heterophylla*
1949	West Virginia	sugar maple *Acer saccharum*
1949	Wisconsin	sugar maple *Acer saccharum*
1947	Wyoming	plains cottonwood *Populus sargentii*

bibliography

BOOKS

Adams, Francis V., M.D. The Asthma Sourcebook: Everything You Need to Know. Los Angeles: Lowell House; 1995. 206 p.

Benson, Lyman; Darrow, Robert A. Trees and Shrubs of the Southwestern Deserts. 3rd. rev. ed. Tuscon (AZ): University of Arizona Press; 1981. 416 p.

Brockman, C. Frank. Trees of North American: A Field Guide to the Major Native and Introduced Species North of Mexico. Zim, Herbert S., editor. New York: Golden Press; 1986. 280 p.

Brown, Lauren. The Audubon Society Nature Guides: Grasslands. New York: Chanticleer Press, Inc.; 1989. 606 p.

Burrill, Larry C.; Dewey, Steven A.; Cudney, David W.; Nelson, B.E.; Lee, Richard D.; Parker, Robert. Weeds of the West. Whitson, Tom D., editor. Newark (CA): The Western Society of Weed Science in Cooperation with the West United States Land Grant Universities Cooperative Extension Services; 1992. 630 p.

Carter, Jack L. Trees and Shrubs of Colorado. Boulder (CO): Johnson Books Distributor; 1988. 165 p.

Collingwood, G.H.; Bruch, Warren D. Knowing Your Trees. Butcher, Devereux, editor. Washington (D.C.): American Foresty Association; 1964. 349 p.

Cunningham, Bill. Montana Wildlands: From Northwest Peaks to Deadhorse Badlands. Helena (MT): American Geo graphic Publishing; 1990. 104 p.

Despain, Don G. Yellowstone Vegetation: Consequences of Environment and History in a Natural Setting. Boulder (CO): Roberts Rinehart, Inc. Publishers; 1990. 239 p.

Duft, Joseph F.; Moseley, Robert K. Alpine Wildflowers of the Rocky Mountains. Missoula (MT): Mountain Press Publishing Company; 1989. 196 p.

Elias, Thomas S. Field Guide to North American Trees. Dambury (CT): Grolier Book Clubs, Inc.; 1989. 948 p.

Engel-Wilson, Carolyn. Landscaping for Desert Wildlife: Trees & Shrubs, Cacti & Succulents, Flowers & Grasses. Phoenix (AZ): Arizona Game & Fish Heritage Fund; 1992. 17 p.

Faber, Phyllis M.; Holland, Robert F. Common Riparian Plants of California: A Field Guide for the Layman. Mill Valley (CA): Pickleweed Press; 1988. 139 p.

Gaines, Xerpha M.; Swan, D.G. Weeds of Eastern Washington and Adjacent Areas. Spokane (WA): Camp-Na-Bor-Lee Association, Inc.; 1972. 349 p.

Grant, John A.; Grant, Carol L. Trees and Shrubs for Pacific Northwest Gardens. 2nd ed. Portland (OR): Timber press; 1990. 456 p.

Harlow, William M., Ph.D.; Harrar, Ellwood S., Ph.D., Sc.D.; White, Fred M. Textbook of Dendrology: Covering the Important Forest Trees of the United States and Canada. 6th ed. New York: McGraw-Hill Book Company; 1979. 510 p.

Hitchcock, C. Leo; Cronquist, Arthur. Flora of the Pacific Northwest: An Illustrated Manual. Seattle (WA): University of Washington Press; 1973. 730 p.

Hoyt, Roland Stewart. Check Lists for Ornamental Plants of Subtropical Regions: A Handbook for Reference. Pacific Palisades (CA): Livingston; 1958. 484 p.

Intermountain Allergy and Asthma Clinic. 1989 Pollen Count. Murray (UT): Intermountain Allergy and Asthma Clinic; 1989. 1 p.

Jackson, Philip L.; Kimerling, A. Jon. Atlas of the Pacific Northwest. 8th ed. Corvallis (OR): Oregon State University Press; 1993. 152 p.

Johnson, Carl M. Native Trees of the Intermountain Region. Logan (UT): Utah State University Cooperative Extension Service; 1984. 82 p.

Kruckeberg, A.R. Gardening with Native Plants of the Pacific Northwest. [place unknown]: University of Washington Press; 1982. 252 p.

Lamb, Samuel H. Woody Plants of the Southwest: A Field Guide with Descriptive Text, Drawing, Range Maps and Photographs. Santa Fe (NM): Sunstone Press; 1989. 177 p.

Lenz, Lee W.; Dourley, John. California Native Trees & Shrubs: For Garden and Environment use in Southern California and Adjacent Areas. Claremont (CA): Rancho Santa Ana Botanic Garden; 1981. 231 p.

MacMahon, James. The Audubon Society Nature Guides: Deserts. New York: Chanticleer Press, Inc.; 1988. 638 p.

Martin, Alexander C. Weeds. New York: Golden Press; 1987. 160 p.

Mathews, Daniel. Cascade-Olympic Natural History. Portland (OR): Raven Editions; 1988. 623 p.

McClintock, Elizabeth, Ph.D.; Halde, Carlyn, Ph.D. Hay Fever Plants of the San Francisco Bay Area. San Francisco (CA): American Lung Association of San Francisco; [date unknown]. 3 p.

McPhee, Marnie. Western Oregon: Portrait of the Land and Its People. Helena (MT): American Geographic Publishing; 1987. 103 p. (Oregon Geographic Series; 2).

McPherson, E. Gregory; Graves, Gregory H. Ornamental and Shade Trees for Utah: A Tree Guide for Intermountain Communities. Logan (UT): Cooperative Extension Services, Utah State University; 1984. 144 p.

Mozingo, Hugh. Shrubs of the Great Basin: A Natural History. Reno (NV): University of Nevada Press; 1987. 342 p.

National Audubon Society. American Wildlife & Plants: A Guide to Wildlife Food Habits. New York: Alfred A. Knopf, Inc.

National Audubon Society. Field Guide to North American Trees: Eastern Region. New York: Alfred A. Knopk, Inc.

Munz, Philip A.; Keck, David A. A California Flora. Berkeley: University of California Press; 1968. 1593 p.

National Xeriscape Council. Xeriscape Gardens: Plants for the Desert Southwest. 3rd ed. Phoenix (AZ): Arizona Municipal Water Users Association; 1991. 30 p.

Preston, Richard J. Jr. North American Trees: A Handbook Designed for Field Use, with Plates and Distribution Maps. 3rd ed. Ames (Iowa): Iowa State University Press; 1977. 397 p.

Reese, Rick. Greater Yellowstone: The National Park and Adjacent Wildlands. Helena (MT): Montana Magazine, Inc.; 1984. 104 p. (Montana Geographic Series; 6).

Sailing, Ann. The Great Northwest Nature Factbook: Remarkable Animals, Plants & Natural Features in Washington, Oregon, Idaho & Montana. Anchorage (AK): Alaska Northwest Books; 1991. 198 p.

Sands, Anne, editor. Riparian Forests in California: Their Ecology and Conservation. Proceedings of the symposium; 1977 May 14; Davis, CA. Davis: The Regents of the University of California; 1980. 122 p. Symposium sponsored by the Institute of Ecology, University of California Davis and the Davis Audubon Society. Originally published as the Institute of Ecology Publication No. 15.

Sargent, Charles S. Manual of Trees of North America. 2nd ed. vol 1. New York: Dover Publications, Inc.: 1965. 455 P.

Sargent, Charles S. Manual of Trees of North America. 2nd ed. vol 2. New York: Dover Publications, Inc.: 1965. 921 p.

Shigo, Alex L. Tree Pruning: A Worldwide Photo Guide. Durham (NH): Shigo and Trees, Associates; 1989. 186 p.

Sinclair, Wayne A.; Lyon, Howard H.; Johnson, Warren T. Diseases of Trees and Shrubs. London: Cornell University Press; 1987. 575 p.

Smith & Hawken. The Book on Outdoor Gardening. New York: Workman Publishing: 1996. 513 p.

Subak-Sharpe, Genell J., editor. Home Health Handbook. [place unknown]: IMP BV/IMP Inc.; 1989. Chapter 3, Heart, Lungs and Blood, Card 15, Asthma.

Subak-Sharpe, Genell J., editor. Home Health Handbook. [place unknown]: IMP BV/IMP Inc.; 1989. Chapter 3, Heart, Lungs and Blood, Card 16, Asthma, Chronic Severe.

Subak-Sharpe, Genell J., editor. Home Health Handbook. [place unknown]: IMP BV/IMP Inc.; 1989. Chapter 9, Special Concerns of Children, Card 3, Asthma Acute.

Subak-Sharpe, Genell J., editor. Home Health Handbook. [place unknown]: IMP BV/IMP Inc.; 1989. Chapter 9, Special Concerns of Children, Card 4, Asthma, Allergic.

Sullivan, William L. Exploring Oregon's Wild Areas: A Guide for Hikers, Backpackers, Climbers, xc Skiers & Paddlers. Seattle (WA): The Mountaineers; 1988. 275 p.

Sunset Books and Sunset Magazine. National Garden Book. Menlo Park (CA): Sunset Books; 1997. 656 p.

Sunset Books and Sunset Magazine. Trees and Shrubs. Menlo Park (CA): Sunset Publishing Corporation; 1993. 144 p.

Sunset Books and Sunset Magazine. Western Garden Book. Menlo Park (CA): Sunset Publishing Corporation; 1988. 592 p.

Taylor, Ronald J. Northwest Weeds: The Ugly and Beautiful Villains of Fields, Gardens, and Roadsides. Missoula (MT): Mountain Press Publishing Company; 1990. 177 p.

U. S. Agricultural Research Service. Common Weeds of the United States. New York: Dover Publications; 1971. 463 p.

Watts, May Theilgard; Watts, Tom. Desert Tree Finder: A Pocket Manual for Identifying Desert Trees. Berkeley (CA): Nature Study Guide; 1974. 61 p.

Watts, Tom. Pacific Coast Tree Finder: A Pocket Manual for Identifying Pacific Coast Trees. Berkeley (CA): Nature Study Guide; 1973. 61 p.

Watts, Tom. Rocky Mountain Tree Finder: A Pocket Manual for Identifying Rocky Mountain Trees. Berkeley (CA): Nature Study Guide; 1972. 61 p.

Welsh, Stanley L. Flowers of the Canyon Country. Moab (UT): Canyonlands National History Association; 1986. 85 p.

Whitman, Ann H., editor. Familiar Trees of North America: Western Region. New York: Alfred A. Knopf, Inc.; 1988. 192 p.

Whitney, Stephen R. A Field Guide to the Cascades and Olympics. Seattle (WA): The Mountaineers; 1983. 288 p.

Whitson, Tom D.; Dewey, Steven A.; Ferrell, Mark A.; Evans, John O.; Miller, Stephen D.; Shaw, Richard J. Weeds and Poisonous Plants of Wyoming and Utah. Whitson, Tom D., editor. Logan (UT): University of Wyoming, Cooperative Extension Services and Utah State University Cooperative Extension Service and Agricultural Experiment Station; 1987. 280 p.

Wodehouse, Roger P., Ph. D. Hayfever Plants: Their Appearance, Distribution, Time of Flowering, and Their Role in Hayfever. 2nd rev. ed. New York: Hafner Publishing Company; 1971. 280 p.

Bibliography

Wuerthner, George. Oregon Mountain Ranges. Helena (MT): American Geographic Publishing; 1987. 104 p. (Oregon Geographic Series; 1).

Zellerbach, Merla. The Allergy Sourcebook: Everything You Need to Know. Los Angeles: Lowell House; 1995. 246 p.

JOURNALS

Bailey, William C., Higgins, Darlene M., Richards, Bonnie M.: Richards, James M. Asthma Severity: A Factor Analytic Investigation. Am J Med 1992 Sep; 93 (9): 263-269

Bernstein, Jonathan A. Occupational Asthma. Postgrad Med 1992 Sep 1; 92(3) : 109-112, 117-118.

Gergen, Peter J.; Weiss, Kevin B. Changing Patterns of Asthma Hospitalization Among Children: 1979 to 1987. JAMA 1990 Oct; 264 (13): 1688-1692

Gorman, Chrisine. Asthma: Deadly...But Treatable. Time 1992 Jun 22; 139 (25): 61-62.

Jaroff, Leon. Allergies: Nothing to Sneeze At. Time 1992 Jun 22; 139 (25): 54-59

Larsen, Gary L. Asthma In Children. N Engl J. Med 1992 Jun; 326 (23): 1540-1545.

Leff, Michael, editor. Treating the Real Cause of Asthma Attacks. Consum Rep Health 1992 Oct; 4 (10): 76-77.

Rumbak, Mark J.; Self, Timothy H. A Diagnostic Approach to "Difficult" Asthma. Postgrad Med 1992 Sep 1; 92(3): 80-86, 89-91.

Schwartz, Leslie. Wheeze Easy. Shape 1996 Mar; 15(7):36-39.

Self, Timothy H.; Rumbak, Mark J,; Kelso, Tiffany M. Correct Use of Metered-Dose Inhalers and Spacer Dividers. Postgrad Med 1992 Sep 1; 92(3); 95-95, 99-103, 106.

Weiss, Kevin B. Seasonal Trends in US Asthma Hospitalizations and Mortality. JAMA 1990 May; 263 (17):2323-2328.

Weiss, Kevin B.; Wagener, Diane K. Changing Patterns of Asthma Mortality: Identifying Target Population at High Risk JAMA 1990 Oct; 264 (13): 1683-1687.

SCIENTIFIC REPORTS

Anderson, Bernice A. Desert Plants of Utah. Logan (UT): Utah Cooperative Extension Service and the U.S. Dept. of Agriculture; [date unknown]. Report No.: EC 376. 146 p. Available from: Utah Cooperative Extension Service, Utah State University, Logan, Utah.

Anderson, Bernice A. Mountain Plants of Northeastern Utah. Logan (UT): Utah Cooperative Extension Services and the U.S. Dept. of Agriculture; 1985 Oct. Circular No.: 319. 149 p. Available from: Utah Cooperative Extension Services, Utah State University, Logan, Utah.

Ballow, Thomas W.; Jones, Bernard M. 1991-1992 Nevada Agricultural Statistics. Reno (NV): U.S. Department of Agriculture and National Agricultural Statistics Service; 1992 Sep. 48 p. Available from: Nevada Agricultural Statistics, Reno, Nevada.

Ballow, Thomas W.; Jones, Bernard M. 1994 Nevada Agricultural Statistics. Reno (NV): U.S. Department of Agriculture - National Agricultural Statistics Service; 1994 Sep. 42 p. Available from: Nevada Agricultural Statistics Service, Reno, Nevada.

Ballow, Thomas W.; Jones, Bernard M. 1992-1993 Nevada Agricultural Statistics. Reno (NV): Nevada Agricultural Statistics Service; 1993 Sep. 44 p. Available from: Nevada Agricultural Statistics Service, Reno, Nevada.

Ballow, Thomas W.; Jones, Bernard M. 1988 and 1989 Nevada Agricultural Statistics. Reno (NV): U.S. Department of Agriculture - National Agricultural Statistics Service; 1989 Sep. 44 p. Available from Nevada Agricultural Statistics, Reno, Nevada.

Bloyd, Barry L.; Kenerson, Debra K. 1991 Arizona Agricultural Statistics Service, Bulletin S-27. Phoenix (AZ): Arizona Agricultural Statistics Service; 1992 Aug. 111 p. Available from: Arizona Agricultural Statistics Service, Phoenix, Arizona.

Bloyd, Barry L.; Bennett, Norman W. 1988 Arizona Agricultural Statistics. Phoenix (AZ): Arizona Agricultural Statistics Service; 1989 Jul. 110 p. Available from: Arizona Agriculture Statistics Service, Phoenix, Arizona.

Coulter, Richard; Thorson, Jerry. 1993 Wyoming Agricultural Statistics. Cheyenne (WY): U.S. Department of Agriculture - National Agricultural Statistics Services; [date unknown]. 98 p. Available from: Wyoming Agricultural Statistics Services.

Coulter, Richard; Thorson, Jerry. 1992 Wyoming Agricultural Statistics. Cheyenne (WY): Wyoming Agriculture Statistics Service; [date unknown]. 99 p. Available from: Wyoming Agriculture Statistics Services.

Coulter, Richard; Thorson, Jerry. 1994 Wyoming Agricultural Statistics. Cheyenne (WY): U.S. Department of Agriculture - National Agricultural Statistics Service; [date unknown]. 98 p. Available from: Wyoming Agricultural Statistics Service.

Fernald, Merritt Lyndon. Gray's Manual of Botany; eighth ed. New York: American Book Company; 1950. 1632 p.

Fitzgerald, Tonie; Notske, Diane; Stone, Melissa; McCrea, Sydney; Gates, Anne. Landscape Plants for the Inland Northwest. Pullman (WA): Washington State Cooperative Extension and the U.S. Department of Agriculture; 1991 Apr. Report No.: EB 1579. 70 p. Available from: Washington State Cooperative Extension, Pullman, Washington.

Franklin, Jerry F.; Dyrness, C.T. Natural Vegetation of Oregon and Washington. Portland: Pacific
Northwest Forest and Range Experiment Station; 1973. USDA Forest Service General Technical Report No.: PNW-8. 417 p. Available from: Pacific Northwest Forest and Range Experiment Station, Portland, Oregon.

Gerhardt, Donald G.; Stringer, Margaret L. 1992 Idaho Agricultural Statistics. Boise (ID): Idaho Agricultural Statistics Service; [date unknown]. 72 p. Available from: Idaho Agricultural Statistics Service, Boise, Idaho.

Gerhardt, Donald G.; Stringer, Margaret L. 1993 Idaho Agricultural Statistics. Boise (ID): Idaho Agricultural Statistics Service; [date unknown]. 76 p. Available from: Idaho Agricultural Statistics Service, Boise, Idaho.

Giacometto, Leo; Bay, Donald M. 1992-1993 Montana Agricultural Statistics. Helena (MT): Montana Agricultural Statistics Service; 1994 Oct. 97 p. Available from: Montana Agricultural Statistics Service, Helena, Montana.

Gneiting, Del Roy J.; Albert, Roland. 1993 Utah Agricultural Statistics. Salt Lake City (UT): Utah Agricultural Statistics Service; [date unknown]. 139 p. Available from: Utah Agricultural Statistics Service, Salt Lake City, Utah.

Gneiting, Del Roy J.; Anderson, Carter D. 1989 Utah Agricultural Statistics. Salt Lake City (UT): Utah Agricultural Statistics Service; [date unknown]. 124 p. Available from: Utah Agricultural Statistics Service, Salt Lake City, Utah.

Gore, Charles E.; Wilken, William M. 1992 New Mexico Agricultural Statistics. Las Cruces (NM): U.S. Department of Agriculture and New Mexico Agricultural Statistics Service; [date unknown]. 72 p. Available from: New Mexico Agricultural Statistics Service, Las Cruces, New Mexico.

Gore, Charles E.; Wilken, William W. 1991 New Mexico Agricultural Statistics. Las Cruces (NM): U.S. Department of Agriculture - New Mexico Agricultural Statistics Service; [date unknown]. 72 p. Available from: New Mexico Agricultural Statistics Services.

Gore, Charles E.; Wilken, William W. 1990 New Mexico Agricultural Statistics. Las Cruces (NM): U.S. Department of Agriculture - New Mexico Agricultural Statistics Service; [date unknown]. 72 p. Available from: New Mexico Agricultural Statistics Service.

Hasslen, Douglas A.; McCall, Jerry. 1991-1993 Washington Agricultural Statistics. Olympia (WA): Washington Agricultural Statistics Service; [data unknown]. 122 p. Available from: Washington Agricultural Statistics, Olympia, Washington.

Hudson, Charles M.; Fretwell, Lance A. Colorado Agricultural Statistics 1990 Preliminary - 1989 Revised Report; Lakewood (CO): Colorado Agricultural Statistics Service; 1991 Jul. 96 p. Available from: Colorado Agricultural Statistics Service, Lakewood, Colorado.

Hudson, Charles M.; Fretwell, Lance A. Colorado Agricultural Statistics 1992 Preliminary - 1991 Revised and Annual Report 1992-1993 Colorado Department of Agriculture; Lakewood (CO): Colorado Agricultural Statistics Service; 1993 Jul. 119 p. Available from: Colorado Agricultural Statistics Service, Lakewood, Colorado.

Hudson, Charles M.; Fretwell, Lance A. Colorado Agricultural Statistics 1993 Preliminary - 1992 Revised and Annual Report 1993-1994 Colorado Department of Agriculture. Lakewood (CO): Colorado Agricultural Statistics Service; 1994 Jul. 119 p. Available from: Colorado Agricultural Statistics Service, Lakewood, Colorado.

Lacey, John R.; Lacey, Celestine A. Controlling Pasture and Range Weeds in Montana. Bozeman (MT): Extension Service, Montana State University and the U.S. Department of Agriculture; [date unknown]. 34 p. Available from: Montana State University, Bozeman, Montana.

Liberty Hyde Bailey Hortorium. Hortus Third: A Concise Dictionary of Plants Cultivated in the United States and Canada. New York: Macmillian Publishing Company, Inc.: 1976. 1290 p.

Mosher, Milton M.; Lunnum, Knut. Trees of Washington. Pullman (WA): Cooperative Extension, College of Agriculture & Home Economics, Washington State University; [date unknown]. Report No.: EB 0440. 41 p. Available from: Cooperative Extension, Washington State University, Pullman, Washington.

Robbins, W.W.; Bellue, Margaret, K.; Ball, Walter S. Weeds of California. Sacramento: State of California, Dept. of Agriculture; [date unknown]. 547 p. Available from: Documents and Publications, Sacramento, California.

Bibliography

Sands, James K.; Lund, Curtis E. 1993 Montana Agricultural Statistics. Helena (MT): Montana Agricultural Statistics Services. 1993 Oct. 97 p. Available from: Montana Agricultural Statistics Service, Helena, Montana.

Stringer, Peggy; Lund, Curtis E. 1995 Montana Agricultural Statistics. Helena (MT): U.S. Department of Agriculture - National Agricultural Statistics Service; 1995 Oct. 160 p. Available from: Montana Agricultural Service, Helena, Montana.

Sutton, Richard; Johnson, Craig W. Landscape Plants from Utah's Mountains. Logan (UT): Cooperative Extension Service, Publications, Utah State University; 1990. Report No.: EC 368. 135 p. Available from: Cooperative Extension Service, Utah State University, Logan, Utah.

Tippett, Jim; Nelson, Dwaine. 1994 California Agriculture Statistics. Sacramento (CA): California Agricultural Statistics Service; 1995 Sep. 96 p. Available from: California Agricultural Statistics Service, Sacramento, California.

U.S. Department of Health and Human Services - National Institutes of Health. Facts About Asthma. Washington (D.C.): U.S. Government Printing Office; 1990 Oct. National Institutes of Health Publication No.: 90-2339. 7p. Available from: National Asthma Education Program Information Center, Bethesda, Maryland.

U.S. Forest Service. Range plant handbook. Washington: U.S. Dept. of Commerce; [date unknown]. Report No.: PB 168-589. 519 p. Available from: Clearinghouse for Federal Scientific and Technical Information, Washington, D.C.

Williams, Paul M.; Kriesel, Ronald F. 1992-1993 Oregon Agriculture & Fisheries Statistics. Salem (OR): Oregon Department of Agriculture; [date unknown]. 83 p. Available from: Oregon Department of Agriculture.

MISCELLANEOUS REFERENCES

1994 Arizona Nursery Association - Retail Directory and Map. Tucson (AZ): Arizona Nursery Association; 1994. 4 p.

Arizona State University Arboretum Guide. Phoenix (AZ): Arizona State University; 1992. 6 p.

Asthma. Fresno (CA): American Lung Association of Central California; 1983. 7 p.

Breckenridge, Patti Hamer. Landscape Plants: A Manual for the Identification of Plant Material. San Luis Obispo, (CA): Patti Hamer Breckenridge; 1984. Desert Botanical Garden: Where the Desert Comes to Life. Phoenix (AZ): Salt River Project; [date unknown]. 9 p.

Hay Fever. San Francisco (CA): American Lung Association of San Francisco; 1986. 4 p.

Hayes, H.D. Tucson Pollen and Mould Calendar. Tucson (AZ): Tucson Clinic, P.C.; [date unknown], 1 p.

Hendrickson, Dianna. Sneezeless Landscaping. San Francisco (CA): American Lung Association; 1989. 3 p.

McClintock, Elizabeth, Ph.D.; Halde, Carlyn, Ph.D. Hay Fever Plants of the San Francisco Bay Area. San Francisco (CA): American Lung Association; [date unknown]. 3 p.

Rotary Pollen Allergy Committee. Fresno's Sneezeless Garden - Reducing Allergy Pollen Is...Nothing to Sneeze At!; [date unknown], 2 p. Available from: Rotary Clubs of Fresno and Clovis, Fresno, California.

Ziering, William H., M.D. Letter to Scott Seargeant. 20 February 1987.

glossary

Glossary

Accent: A plant or plants that compliment a landscape by contrasting or standing out.

Acidic/Acid soil: A soil with a pH value below 7.0. Soil pH is determined by the ratio of hydrogen to hydroxyl ions. Many plants need a acidic soil to grow their best or survive. Some elements are more available to plants at a acidic level.

Alkaline/Basic soil: A soil with a pH value above 7.0. A soil pH is determined by the ratio of hydrogen to hydroxyl ions. Western soils tend to have higher pH values than soils in the east.

Allergen: Any substance that produces an allergic reaction.

Allergy: An exaggerated or abnormal reaction to a substances, situations or physical states harmless to most people.

Allergist: A doctor specializing in the treatment of allergy.

Allergenic: Causing an allergic reaction.

Annual: A plant that completes its life cycle in one year or less and dies.

Anthers: The pollen-bearing portion of the stamen

Antibody: Molecules produced by the body to fight foreign substances.

Antihistamine: Medication taken to counteract the effects of histamine which is produced by the body when exposed to an allergen.

Aphid: Tiny soft bodied insect that sucks the sap from plants and secretes a shiny, sticky substance called honeydew. Aphids belong to the Homoptera order of insects which includes scale, whiteflies, leafhoppers, etc.

Architect: A person licensed to plan and design buildings, homes and living spaces.

Aromatic: A pleasant fragrant plant that can be smelled from a distance.

Asthma: A condition whereby the bronchial tubes are obstructed usually by an allergen causing the person to have shortness of breath, wheezing, coughing.

Atopic: Anyone who possess the capacity to become symptomatic (allergic).

Avoidance: A practice of staying away from the allergens that cause a person to become symptomatic.

Allergy Free Living: A book on allergy prevention through education and active participation by the allergy sufferer (and others) to remove the plants that are allergy producing and replace them with allergy free plants or low pollen producers in the three main places we spend 90 percent of our time: home, work, and surrounding community.

Background Plant: A plant of sufficient size and shape that under normal circumstances should be planted in the rear, perimeter or behind all other plants.

Basal Stalks: Leaves that originate from the base instead of a branch or trunk.

Birds and the Bees: A phrase or icon indicating the relationship between these organisms and the allergy-free plants they pollinate.

Bonsai: An oriental art of dwarfing trees or shrubs by planting in very small containers and consistently and selectivly pruning them.

Botanical Name: The scientific name given to each plant that properly identifies them anywhere in the world. No two plants have the same botanical name. These names are in the Latin language.

Broadleaf:	A term describing a general leaf characteristic of plants that have a determinable midrib and some amount of width to their leaves. Compared to needles or scales of other plants.
Certified Arborist:	A person licensed in professional tree care, not just tree trimming.
Chlorotic:	A element deficient plant or part of a plant exhibiting yellowish foliage which are normally green. Iron is one of the elements missing in a plants "diet" that cause chlorosis. High pH can cause chlorosis especially in plants that like neutral or acidic soil.
Chronic:	A repeated, recurring or habitual disease description.
Clusters:	Leave or flowers grouped together that originate from one central area.
Common Name:	The laymen name for each plant. There can be several common names for a plant or several plants can have the same common name.
Compound Leaf:	Several to many leaflets attached to a secondary leaf stock or (petiolule) which is attached to the main leaf stock (petiole) which is attached to the stem or branch.
Conical:	Cone shaped. Pyramidal.
Conifer:	Referring to cone bearing trees like pine trees.
Container Plant:	A root system that can grow in a limited or confined space (container) and still maintain an attractive healthy look for several to many years.
Cosmopolitan plant:	A plant that is found almost everywhere, especially in populated areas.
Cultivar:	A horticultural variety that was created and continues to be used under cultivation. They are distinguished by having a third botanical name in single quotes of not more than three words. Abelia grandiflora 'Edward Goucher'. The 'Edward Goucher' denotes a cultivar.
Cut Flower:	A flower that can be removed from a plant and used in decorative or floral arrangement and keeps its beauty for a variable but limited time.
Deciduous:	A process or condition whereby some plants loose all their leaves in preparation for rest. This is usually in the fall and winter. However, a small number of plants are summer deciduous.
Deep Rooted Tree:	A tree who root system that tends to grow semi-vertically into the ground or at lower levels in the soil so as not to disturb or ruin nearby planted objects, i.e sidewalks, foundations.
Desensitization:	Processes to reduce allergy symptoms. They can be medical or preventative.
Double Flower:	Flowers with a second layer, row or whorl of petals.
Drought Resistant:	A plant that can survive without supplemental water for long periods or seasons.
East:	A loosely used term meaning states east of and including Michigan to Louisiana.
Elliptical:	Leaves that are oblong but have narrow or rounded ends. The leaf is widest near the middle.
Environment:	Where you live; home, work, and surrounding community.
Established:	A plant that has acclimated to its new home or environment.
Evergreen:	A condition where a plant retains the majority of its leaves all year long. These trees do drop leaves. It is usually throughout the year. Some evergreens are actually messier than some deciduous plants.
Exposure:	A term indicating the amount of sun a plant will receive during the daylight hours.

Glossary

Fascicles: Dense cluster or bundle. As in pine needles.

Fast Growth: In trees it usually means growth (mass) of 4' or more per year. In shrubs it usually means over 3' per year.

Female Flower: The part of the flower that produces the reproductive seed of the plant.

Filler Plant: A plant or plants that are used in many situations to lessen the voids in the landscape or "fill" certain areas that may appear to be bare or needing something.

Fire Retardant: The ability of a plant to withstand a fire without appreciable damage.

Fire Blight: A serious disease of plants in the rose family. Fire blight is caused by a bacteria and infects plants through openings in the flowers.

Flower Spikes: A stock on which flowers appear. They are usually in an upright position.

Foot Traffic: A term meaning the amount or duration a plant (usually ground cover) can withstand being walked on without damaging the plants appearance or causing necrosis (death).

Formal Hedge: Usually a shrub that is pruned into geometric shapes and maintained in those shapes. Mostly used in association with formal landscapes.

Frequent Water: Watering plants three or more times per week.

Frond: The leaf of a fern or palm.

Full Sun: A plant that will grow or thrive in areas without shade.

Good Drainage: Soil that will not hold standing water for more than 4 to 8 hours.

Ground Cover   A low growing plant used to sufficiently cover bare flat or slopped ground. The plant(s) root system must also be capable of retarding soil erosion.

Growth Rate: The amount of mass a plant displays over a given period usually one year.

Gulf States: The states that have ocean fronts along the Gulf of Mexico. These are eastern Texas, Louisiana, Alabama, Mississippi and Florida.

Herb: A plant that doesn't contain true wood or is mostly without true wood. They are softer tissued plants. Sometimes referred to plants with medicinal properties.

High Water: Plants that need large quantities and or applications of water three or more times per week.

Histamine: A substance released by the body in response to an allergen. This can lead to allergy symptoms.

Hybrid Cross: A plant created from the cross pollination of two different species.

Hypersensitivity: Exhibiting allergenic reactions.

Immune System: The bodies way of fighting or resisting diseases.

Inconspicuous: Flower parts that are not easily seen or a plant grown for characteristics other than flowering.

Infection: Intrusion of the body by a harmful microorganism. The transfer of energy from the host to the pathogen.

Infertile Soil: Soils that are low or lack certain elements needed to sustain most plant life. A few plants can grow in these soil conditions.

Informal Hedge:	Usually a shrub that is not pruned or is selectively pruned to keep its natural form or shape.
Invasive Roots:	Roots that are very aggressive and usually grow near the soil surface causing many problems with man made structures including sidewalks, curbs, sewer systems, and some foundations.
Inhalant:	Particles light enough to stay afloat in the air to potentially be taken into the respiratory system (lungs).
Irritant:	Substances that can cause anyone to have inflamation or become symptomatic.
Juvenile Leaves:	Adolescent leaves. They are different in shape and size.
Lanceolate:	Lance shaped leaves.
Landscape Architect:	A person licensed to plan and design exterior environments or landscapes.
Lawn Substitute:	Plants (usually ground covers) that are used in place of traditional lawn grasses. An example is dichondra.
Leaf Burn:	Dead areas on a leaf, usually caused by lack of water, high salt content, over fertilizing or infection.
Leaf Margin:	The edge of a leaf.
Leaf Spot:	A dead roundish area on a leaf usually caused by a pathogen or insect.
Leggyness:	A plant that has grown past the point of being compact. Overgrown with very little interior foliage.
Locally Common:	A plant that is found in most urban and rural areas or regions within the United States.
Low Water:	A plant that only needs supplemental water once or twice a month during times of no natural water (rain, etc.).
Male Flower:	The part of a flower that produces pollen.
Mass Planting:	Plants of the same species planted closely together in a specific area by themselves or in association with other plants of the same arrangement.
Midrib:	The center vein in a leaf.
Midwest:	A loosely used term meaning States in the central part of the United States from Wisconsin and North Dakota to Oklahoma and Arkansas.
Mildew:	A cottony usually whitish coating on leaves and other things caused by a fungal organism.
Moderate Growth:	In trees, it arbitrarily means 2' to 4' of growth or mass (not necessarily just in height) produced in one year. In shrubs it arbitrarily means 1' to 3' of growth or mass produced in one year.
Moderate Water:	A plant that needs supplemental water at least once per week but not more than twice a week during times of no natural water (rain, etc.)
Monoecious:	Male and female flower parts on the same plant.
Multi-Trunk:	A tree that has more than one main stem originating from or close to the base.
Natural Areas:	Areas within the United States that have not been disturbed by man in regards to the native vegetation.

Glossary

Naturalized: A plant that is not endemic or native to the United States but has established itself in certain areas to a point where it can reproduce and compete successfully with existing plant material without the aid of man.

Needle: The leaf of a conifer.

Nematode: A microscopic unisegmented worm that is parasitic to plant roots and lives in the soil.

New Wood: Growth (wood) that is produced in the spring. This usually is a characteristic that determines when to prune a tree or shrub to promote flowering and or fruit.

Night Lighting: Lighting systems specially designed to illuminate and accent landscape situations. They are usually low voltage.

Oak Root Fungus: Usually in reference to Armillaria mellea, a fungus that attacks the root system of many plants including oaks.

Oblong: Leaves longer than wide, usually with parallel sides.

Old Fashion Gardens: Gardens or landscapes indicative of the past. They are usually in association with certain plants rather than landscape features, i.e. roses, gardenias, hydrangeas.

Ornamental Plant: Plants that almost entirely grow in urban and rural man made landscapes. Plants that are not abundant in nature.

Oval: Broadly elliptic about 1-1/2 times as long as wide with rounded ends.

Partial Shade: Plants that need some shade during the sunlight hours usually in the afternoon but can be anytime.

Perennial: A plant that survives more than three years but usually is used in reference to longevity. Year after year.

Petiole: The stalk of a leaf.

pH: A numerical designation of soil and other biological systems acidity or alkalinity based on a scale of 0-14 with 7.0 being neutral.

Phytophora spp: A fungal organism that infects plants.

Pinnate: Leaves or leaflets on either side of the same stock.

Pollen: The male sexual reproductive part of the plant. Pollen from some plants causes allergy symptoms.

Pollution: Anything that contaminates the air, water, food or ourselves.

Pony Pack: Plants (usually flowers) grown in a small container usually 2" by 2".

Post Nasal Drip: A condition where nasal fluids (mucus) flow down the throat and nose often causing soreness or infection.

Prostrate: Plants that grow more horizontally than vertically such as ground cover.

Reseed: Plants that can readily reproduce from seed in many landscape situations without the aid of man.

Resistant: The ability to withstand the effects or action of.

Rhizomes: An underground stem capable of asexual reproduction.

Riparian: Plants that naturally grow in or close to water.

Rock Gardens: Landscapes where the main features are plants and rocks.

Root Rot: The decay of roots by a microorganism. Over watering, and root injury are two main causes.

Roots: An organ of a tree designed to mechanically support, store energy reserves and to gather elements and water from the soil.

Runners: A thin trailing or prostrate shoot growing on top of the ground taking root at the nodes.

Rural: Pertaining to country life or living. People who live in the country.

Selective Pruning: The art and science of pruning only the parts of the tree or shrub that will achieve the intended pruning needs or desires. Pruning with a specific goal in mind.

Serrate: Leaves having a saw-toothed edge.

Shear: Non-selective pruning where the outer leaves are pruned usually into a desired shape. As in formal landscapes.

Simple Leaf: One leaf on a petiole.

Single Flower: Referring to the one whorl of petals on a flower, or referring to one flower.

Skyline Tree: Tall trees with picturesque features that enhance the horizon or they incorporate the sky into the landscape.

Slow Growth: Trees and shrubs that arbitrarily grow 1' per year or less.

Soggy: Soil that is constantly wet and almost saturated.

Sooty Mold: A mold that grows on plant surfaces from the sticky honeydew secretion of Homoptera insects including aphids and scale.

Spathe: A bract or leaf surrounding or subtending a flower cluster or a spadix.

Specimen: A plant(s) that stands out more than all the other plants in the landscape.

Spent Flowers: Flowers that have wilted and withered and are no longer attractive.

Spider Mite: A very tiny spider (not an insect) that damages and or kills plants or plant parts.

Spine: A sharp woody growth from the trunk or stem (thorn-like).

Spp.: Any species within the genera (plural form).

Spring Color: Plants that have showy flowers in the spring.

Stamens: The pollen carrying part of the flower.

Suckers: A shoot growing from below the ground.

Symptomatic: Showing the signs of allergies.

Syringe: Spraying the foliage of a plant with water to cosmetically clean or improve the appearance.

Thrip: Small insects that have rasping-sucking mouth parts and cause a lot of plant damage. Thrip are sometimes vectors of plant viruses.

Glossary

Tolerant: The ability of a plant to endure short term deviations in its environment. A quality some plants possess that allows them to endure changes in their environment that would otherwise severely damage or kill other plants.

Tomentose: A dense covering of short matted, wooly hairs.

Topiary: The art of pruning plants into specific shapes or characters.

Topical: Localized to one area or region.

Trellis: A lattice or similar structure used to grow vines or plants on.

Triggers: A laymen term meaning allergen.

Tubular Flower: A trumpet shaped flower.

Umbel: Many flowers bunched together usually with a flat or slightly rounded top with stocks (pedicels) originating at one basic point. Umbrella-like.

Understory: A situation or condition where a plant is or can grow in the shadow or within the canopy of another larger tree and thrive.

Unpopulated area: Areas where nobody lives or areas where man lives but has not changed or introduced new plants into the area.

Urban: City life. Living in the city.

USDA Climate Zones: Areas plotted on a North American map indicating geographic locations that have similar cold temperatures. This is used to indicate where plants can grow geographically based on minimum temperatures.

Variegated: Leaves or flowers that have at least to different colors.

Veins: The transport vessels in a plant (leaf).

Verticillium Wilt: A disease that disrupts a plants vascular system disabling the transport of water and elements.

Vigorous: A plant that grows extremely fast in either the root system, flowers and or foliage.

Water Sprouts: A fast growing shoot at the base, on the trunk or branches. They usually die within 3 years.

Well-Drained Soils: Soils that have enough porosity to percolate normal amounts of water away leaving a positive ratio of water and gasses in the soil structure.

West: A loose term meaning all 11 western states excluding Texas.

Wheezing: A whistling gasping sound made by some allergy sufferers and asthmatics stemming from their allergic condition. This is an indication the person is having difficulty breathing.

Whorl: A set of three or more flowers, petals, stems or leaves arranged in a circle at their point of attachment.

Woody: Plants that exhibit or have stems or trunks that resemble or contain wood.

index

COMMON NAME

COMMON NAME

BOTANICAL NAMES

BOTANICAL NAMES

PHOTOGRAPHERS AND ILLUSTRATORS

PHOTOGRAPHERS:

Thomas E. Eltzroth: Aloysia triphylla page 29, Symphoicarpus albus 55, Bauhinia variegata (full view) 60, Leptospermum laevigatum (inset) 71, Chamaedorea elegans 75, Pinus thumbergiana 80, Prunus caroliniana 82, Dichondra micrantha 86, Alcea rosea 90, 168 Campanula spp. 91, Cathranthus roseus 91, Dicentra spp. 92, Gladiolus spp. 93, 168 Hemercallis spp. 93, Peony hybridus, 94, Tulipa spp. 95, Zantedeschia spp. 96, Calocedrus decurrens (2) 116, Chamaecyparis lawsoniana (2) 117, Amaranthus spp. (flowers) (2) 150.

Gary Leyrer: Rhododendron spp. 52, Weigela florida 57, Abeis concolor (inset) 58, Abies grandis 58, Cotinus coggygria (full view) 64.

Larry C. Burrill: Dactylis glomerata 142, Holcus lanatus (full view) 143.

Tom Whitson: Holcus lanatus (inset) 143.

Allan Morgan: Hymenoclea spp. (2) 103.

©LECO.: Abies concolor (full view) 58.

Tim Satterfield: Artemisia spp. (full view and upper inset) 98, Atriplex spp. 99, Chrysothamnus spp. 101, Tamarix spp. 132.

Scott E. Seargeant: All other photographs. Photograph equipment provided by Janan and Chuck Miller.

ORNAMENTAL HORTICULTURE CONSULTANT:
Doug Watson

ART DIRECTOR:
Lesley D. Gleason, Lesley & Associates

SENIOR GRAPHIC DESIGNER:
Jeff Marks, Lesley & Associates

MAP ILLUSTRATOR:
Jennifer Manduffie

ABOUT THE AUTHOR

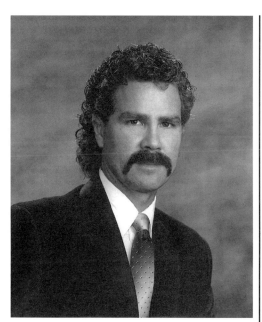

Author Scott E. Seargeant
International Certified Arborist

Scott E. Seargeant earned his Bachelors of Science Degree in Ornamental Horticulture in 1984 from California Polytechnic State University in San Luis Obispo, California. The next twelve years Mr. Seargeant owned and operated Seargeant Landscape & Arboriculture, a full service landscape design, installation, maintenance and tree consulting business.

Presently, Mr. Seargeant specializes in landscape and tree consulting for private and public entities including hospitals, insurance companies, government agencies, and businesses. Mr. Seargeant's career has shifted into the publishing business with a focus still in horticulture. Mr. Seargeant wanted to be able to present his knowledge and experiences to the public on a national and international level. "I felt the best way to communicate my information was through books. So I started Seargeant Publishing Company, Inc. Being President gives me the control I need to present to the public information they need, in its purest form."

Mr. Seargeant has also earned a California Landscape Contractors License, Qualified Applicators License, and an International Certified Arborist license. He was producer and host for five years of Central Valley Gardening, a cable television show on gardening geared for the homeowner.

He has received several awards for his creative landscapes and arboriculture knowledge. Mr. Seargeant received the City of Visalia, (California), " Friends of the Oak Award," for outstanding dedication to the health, safety and preservation of oak trees.

He has consulted for the California Department of Transportation (Cal-Trans) on oak tree identification and survival during highway construction. He has traveled and consulted throughout the Western United States as well as internationally , including a year and a half as the consulting arborist for the Club de Golf, Lomas Golf and Country Club in Mexico City, Mexico. He has consulted for many others, both private and public, including expert witness in court cases.

Closer to home Mr. Seargeant co-chaired the design, installation and funding of the largest allergy-free park in the United States. He continues to lecture and teach others concerning allergies and allergy-free plants. He has written several horticultural articles and pamphlets and is now the author of "The Birds and the Bees Guide to Allergy-Free Living." Seargeant's future titles will cover medical, horticulture and children's educational books.

Replacing Allergy Producing Plants with Allergy-Free Plants

REPLACEMENT PLANT PROJECT SHEET

List Allergy Producing Plants In Your Landscape

List Possible Allergy-Free Plant Substitutions

SHRUBS:

ALLERGY-FREE SHRUBS:

1. _____

  1. _____ 3. _____
  2. _____ 4. _____

2. _____

  1. _____ 3. _____
  2. _____ 4. _____

3. _____

  1. _____ 3. _____
  2. _____ 4. _____

4. _____

  1. _____ 3. _____
  2. _____ 4. _____

5. _____

  1. _____ 3. _____
  2. _____ 4. _____

6. _____

  1. _____ 3. _____
  2. _____ 4. _____

7. _____

  1. _____ 3. _____
  2. _____ 4. _____

8. _____

  1. _____ 3. _____
  2. _____ 4. _____

TREES:

ALLERGY-FREE TREES:

1. _____

  1. _____ 3. _____
  2. _____ 4. _____

2. _____

  1. _____ 3. _____
  2. _____ 4. _____

3. _____

  1. _____ 3. _____
  2. _____ 4. _____

4. _____

  1. _____ 3. _____
  2. _____ 4. _____

5. _____

  1. _____ 3. _____
  2. _____ 4. _____

6. _____

  1. _____ 3. _____
  2. _____ 4. _____

7. _____

  1. _____ 3. _____
  2. _____ 4. _____

8. _____

  1. _____ 3. _____
  2. _____ 4. _____

Replacing Allergy Producing Plants with Allergy-Free Plants

REPLACEMENT PLANT PROJECT SHEET

List Allergy Producing Plants In Your Landscape	**List Possible Allergy-Free Plant Substitutions**

GROUND COVERS:

ALLERGY-FREE GROUND COVERS:

1. _____
   1. _____ 3. _____
   2. _____ 4. _____

2. _____
   1. _____ 3. _____
   2. _____ 4. _____

3. _____
   1. _____ 3. _____
   2. _____ 4. _____

4. _____
   1. _____ 3. _____
   2. _____ 4. _____

5. _____
   1. _____ 3. _____
   2. _____ 4. _____

6. _____
   1. _____ 3. _____
   2. _____ 4. _____

7. _____
   1. _____ 3. _____
   2. _____ 4. _____

8. _____
   1. _____ 3. _____
   2. _____ 4. _____

FLOWERS:

ALLERGY-FREE FLOWERS:

1. _____
   1. _____ 3. _____
   2. _____ 4. _____

2. _____
   1. _____ 3. _____
   2. _____ 4. _____

3. _____
   1. _____ 3. _____
   2. _____ 4. _____

4. _____
   1. _____ 3. _____
   2. _____ 4. _____

5. _____
   1. _____ 3. _____
   2. _____ 4. _____

6. _____
   1. _____ 3. _____
   2. _____ 4. _____

7. _____
   1. _____ 3. _____
   2. _____ 4. _____

8. _____
   1. _____ 3. _____
   2. _____ 4. _____

Creating An Allergy-Free Living Landscape

ALLERGY-FREE PLANT PROJECT SHEET

List Your Favorite Allergy-Free Plants For Your New Landscape Design

SHRUBS:

1. _____
2. _____
3. _____
4. _____
5. _____
6. _____
7. _____
8. _____

GROUND COVERS:

1. _____
2. _____
3. _____
4. _____
5. _____
6. _____
7. _____
8. _____

TREES:

1. _____
2. _____
3. _____
4. _____
5. _____
6. _____
7. _____
8. _____

FLOWERS

1. _____
2. _____
3. _____
4. _____
5. _____
6. _____
7. _____
8. _____

Allergy-Free Living

PERSONAL NOTES

_____
_____
_____
_____
_____
_____
_____

Creating An Allergy-Free Plant Landscape

LANDSCAPE DESIGN PROJECT SHEET

Design Your New Allergy-Free Landscape Before Planting

Design One

Design Two

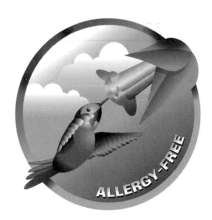

REGISTER YOUR BOOK

To Receive Updates On Allergy-Free Living

And Information About Future Publications From

Seargeant Publishing Company, Inc.

CALL, FAX OR WRITE TO US.

IMPORTANT NUMBERS
Phone: 209-738-8085 • Fax: 209-738-9183

MAILING ADDRESS
Seargeant Publishing Co., Inc.

P.O. Box 1849

Visalia, California 93279

WEBSITE ADDRESS
www.seargeantpublishing.com

REGISTER #_____